# RIGHT SIZING YOUR LIFE

## LOSING 70 LBS.

Monica M. Schmelter

authorHOUSE®

*AuthorHouse™*
*1663 Liberty Drive*
*Bloomington, IN 47403*
*www.authorhouse.com*
*Phone: 1-800-839-8640*

*First published by AuthorHouse 4/28/2009*

*ISBN: 978-1-4389-5851-4 (sc)*
*ISBN: 978-1-4389-5852-1 (hc)*

*Printed in the United States of America*
*Bloomington, Indiana*

*This book is printed on acid-free paper.*

To Barry Campbell, Bobbi Mofield, and Peggy and Johnny Keel

Thank you for all your hard work and mentoring. I appreciate all you taught me and how you taught me to Right Size My Life. When I walked through the doors of Sports Village I was afraid to work out. All of you taught me to face my fears and conquer them. I would never have been able to Right Size My Life without your program "Next Biggest Loser". Your hard work helped me change my life. My deepest appreciation to all of you. Thank you for showing me how to Right Size My Life.
Monica Schmelter

# TABLE OF CONTENTS

Foreward   ix

Introduction   xi

    Right Sizing Your Life How I lost 70 pounds   xi

Reasons Excuses and Other Stuff   1

My Story   4

The First Weigh in "Black Monday"   8

Overview of Months 2 & 3   25

Starting to Work Out   30

All or Nothing Workouts   33

Overview of Months 4 & 5   37

    Slow and Steady Wins the Weight-loss Race   37

    Our Eyes are Bigger Than our Stomachs
    – a lesson in Portion Sizes   39

Overview of Months 6 & 7   54

    The Big Picture is key to RSYL.   57

Overview of Months 8 & 9   64

Overview of Months 10 & 11   71

The Final Four   79

Maintenance   85

RSYL Lifestyle   89

Basic Nutrition   91

    RSYL Food Shopping Tips for basic Meats   92

RSYL Dinner Recipe Ideas   97

RSYL - FAQ's   108

# FOREWARD

Observing Monica over the years has been like watching the average American woman in an effort to be better both physically and mentally. She is your typical gym mom that would quietly slip in, walk the treadmill, and quietly slip out. Monica has always been on of those members that you notice because she is so beautiful and always has a contagious smile and big caring eyes. Yes, Monica is an average American mom trying to be the best she can be, the only way she knows.

I could see her struggle over the years to achieve her fitness goals and become her ideal weight. She would timidly watch what others were doing in the group exercise rooms but, like so many others, was afraid to jump in. Unlike many however, Monica never gave up. She was determined to find a way.

One day she made the scary and tough decision to participate in "the next biggest loser". This was the turning point in her journey to better health, greater confidence, and happiness within.

She learned that she can participate in classes without looking foolish. She learned other areas of the gym were not so scary and intimidating. Monica has become a very confident gym member that is truly an important part of the club. She made it through those difficult years with a relentless attitude and determination.

It gives me joy to see how Monica has become a true advocate for health and an example to all struggling women proving that "you can do it".

She is such a pleasure in the gym with her gentle spirit and heart for Jesus. She approaches wellness with balance and common sense.

In today's world it is very difficult to live a healthy lifestyle. It requires a change of thinking about what and when we eat. Like Monica, once you get over the hump, the rest is easy.

Both Monica and I are passionate about helping you to do it too.

Peggy Keel, Owner

Sports Village Fitness

Lebanon, TN

www.sportsvillagefitness.com

# INTRODUCTION

## RIGHT SIZING YOUR LIFE
## HOW I LOST 70 POUNDS

When I was about 8 or 9 years old I was given the nick name of "Minnesota Fats". I didn't like the name or appreciate the teasing. But that's the way it was.

I was known as the "chubby girl". You know the one that wears the charming ½ sizes from the chubby girl department. The one to whom well meaning people say "oh but you have such a pretty face!" I'm sure you get the idea.

I can remember trying all kinds of diets and exercise to get rid of the problem. Nothing I tried worked. This went on for 43 long years.

At 43 years of age I decided that I would embark on a Right Sizing my Life Journey. I wasn't even sure I could do it. I was just willing to try "one more time". After all I had never been at my goal weight, nor had I ever worked out or participated in any kind of sports.

Nonetheless, I started this weight loss journey with prayer. After 12 months (one long year) of dieting and working out I reached goal weight for the first time in my entire life. It took me an entire year to lose 70 pounds but I did it.

After completing the weight loss journey I started the maintenance phase. I was absolutely astonished that I had no problem in keeping the weight off. The right sizing lifestyle I had embarked on had made all of the difference.

I struggled with writing this book for many reasons. First, it's a personal subject. Second, there is already a lot of really good information out there on health and fitness. What continued to resonate in my mind though was how much easier it would have been for me if I would have had just a "regular person" share with me the good, the bad, and the ugly in their weight loss journey.

Don't get me wrong we need the expert advice and opinions. It's just that there is nothing like learning from someone who has been there. I so much want to help and encourage people because I have been there. I know the struggles. I know the difficulties. Yet I found that it was really just a few habits that separated me from the weight loss and fitness that I had longed for all of my life.

That's why I wrote the book. I want to help others just like me who struggle with weight issues, unhealthy dieting, and can't seem to find the time or motivation to work out. What I found is that it can be done. It won't be easy. It won't be quick. But you can do it. You can lose the weight and keep it off.

# REASONS, EXCUSES AND OTHER STUFF

We live in a culture of supersized combo meals, drive thru's and plus sized portions. Match that with office jobs, sitting in front of a computer all day, and you've got an equation for packing on the pounds. I think we all know the eat less and exercise more solution but most of us have a myriad of excuses on why that just can't happen in real life.

Let's face it eating healthy requires planning ahead. Fast food is convenient. It's a last minute option and while it may be loaded with fat it will stop a stomach from grumbling. So what about the exercise part? Well of course that takes time and energy. Most Americans say they are short on time and oh so tired already. How could we possibly add one more thing to do in our schedule?

Before beginning my own weight loss journey I could never imagine how I could make the time to work out. In fact, I frequently hurried though each and every day. After all here is a list of all my jobs – I am a wife, mom, a full time employee, traveling speaker, and I'm also a leader my local church. My days and evenings were full. I was very tired and with each passing year I was a few pounds heavier.

Despite the weight gain I enjoyed and appreciated my life. I often thought I was too busy and that my schedule was packed with too much stuff, but at the same time, I felt helpless to change it. One day I had a conversation with my boss, Mr. Bob D'Andrea, Founder and President of Christian Television Network. In that conversation I specifically asked him how he found the time to accomplish so much. His answer astounded me and I couldn't get it out of my head. He said, "I don't worry about having enough time to get everything done. God gives me enough time to do everything I need to do". Keep in mind that Mr. D'Andrea is a very accomplished person. In fact, he's accomplished more than anyone I know. He's a pioneer in Christian broadcasting, a businessman and yet he is the most gentle and steadfast leader you could meet. I have the utmost respect for him and he said simply I don't worry about having enough time to get everything done. Perhaps his answer sounds simple but it's also profound. God gives him enough time to do what he needs to do? His answer makes me think and pray.

Since I know that God is no respecter of persons I realize this means that God has also given me enough time to do what I need to do. So why then did I feel so frequently pressed for time? Why the stress, the scramble to get things done? What caused my standard response to be "I am so busy"? Then I realized here I have been rushing through life – looking for more time – feeling like there was always to much to do and my boss who has much more responsibility than me said that God had given him enough time.

His response has continued to resonate in my life. In fact, his response caused me to "Right Size my Life". Instead of being worried about time and trying to rush I started to relax. I prayed each day that God would give me the time and priorities I needed for that day and those assignments. Gradually, I began to see my focus change. It's not that I had less to do necessarily; it's that I approached life with a different perspective.

As I began by faith to relax and pray about my life everything changed. I found myself developing new habits and priorities. Amazingly my over-scheduled life took on a new shape. I still had a lot of responsibilities but they were no longer the ruler of my day. I approached each assignment with faith that all would go well instead of being worried about "running out of time".

In fact, I became so confident that all would go well that I stopped "living on the run". I started spending quiet time in planning my day. I quit planning meetings back to back thinking that was the only way I could get things done. I found more praying and planning helped me have less meetings simply because I was more organized and focused. My mind was calmer and better able to concentrate and delegate.

Right Sizing your Life is based partially on the concept that "less is more". If you think about it Jesus accomplished more than any of us ever will. He accomplished more with less because His Father's Kingdom and priorities were His primary concern. He certainly had opportunities for distractions and confused priorities but He was so focused on our Father He didn't give way to pull of the world's system.

Most of us are running around "short on time" because we're working really hard to make a living, to accomplish something. We are in fact so focused on these areas that most Americans don't take care of themselves. After all, we're too busy working and commuting doing all the things we think it takes to earn a living and be a family.

What if we really believed God's way was best? What if Mr D'Andrea is right? What if God has really given all of us enough time to do what we need to do? What if there is really enough time for you to eat healthily and work out?

All of us have enough time to do what we need to do. It starts by recognizing this fact. Once we build our lives on this foundation of the truth everything else begins to take shape.

# MY STORY

Ever since I can remember I struggled with my weight. In elementary school I was the "chubby girl". I wore those really fun ½ sizes and I hated every minute of it. I hated clothes shopping. I hated summer. I hated swim suits.

The fact is I could never really figure out why I was chubby. It didn't seem like I ate anymore than any other kid my age. But I did weigh more and I did try diets, fitness programs and following others well meaning advice. It's just that none of that really seemed to work for me.

Even when I managed to lose a few pounds I ended up putting them right back on. For me, dieting was synonymous with starving myself. To make matters worse, as far as I was concerned, sports, physical activity, and breaking a sweat, was pretty much out of the question.

My fixation with my weight increased with every passing year. It started in elementary school but it was still with me in high school. I was sure that if I could just lose weight that all of my problems would be solved. Well at least most of my problems anyway. I mean after all doesn't everybody think that thin is better? Aren't thinner people happier? Don't they have more friends? Don't they have more boyfriends? Wouldn't clothes shopping be much easier?

Actually each year I grew more miserable with my weight. I tried to accept being "chubby" – I told myself that is was just my DNA – that's the way it needed to be. For awhile that would work. Then I would get sick of my weight and try another diet. Sure, I would lose some weight. I would usually starve myself. Many times I cut my caloric intake to 500 calories a day. I beamed with pride at my discipline and when people would see the weight loss they would be so thrilled with me and my progress.

The thing about that was I couldn't stay at 500 calories a day for longer than a few months. That's a good thing because it's not healthy. If you've been on starvation diets before you know what I am talking about. You walk around hungry and with a headache. You are lightheaded and on edge. The good news is that the RSYL journey is not about starving. God did not intend for you to starve yourself. The thing about the starvation diets that I learned is that the moment I stopped starving myself I started putting the weight back on and sometimes added a few more pounds too. This set in a frustration and hopeless level that's difficult to describe.

Don't get me wrong, I got many nice compliments along the way. Lots of people told me I was pretty. Even guys told me I was pretty. I did get asked out on dates but still in the back of my mind I wondered why I needed to be "larger" than the ideal standard. I figured the ideal standard to be somewhere around 115 –125 pounds and wearing a size 6. That idea or opinion is definitely reinforced in our culture. The truth is we are all aware that we live in a thin, youth, and beauty oriented culture. The pressure on women (men too) is tremendous. Certainly, that is why eating disorders have grown at such an alarming rate.

When I graduated from high school I was 5 feet and 3 inches and weighed 143 pounds. I was sure no other high school girl in the universe weighed that much. All of my friends wore size 5's and 7's and there I was in a size 11. At the same time, you need to know even though I was overweight I was very concerned with fashion and wearing only the finest of outfits perfectly accesorized. I was never comfortable dressing casually – I dressed up every day and tried to cover up the fact that I was larger than the average young woman my age.

This continued on throughout adulthood. I vacillated between starving and overeating. From never exercising to working out 5 times per week. I lost weight and gained weight. Inside I was miserable. On the outside I smiled a lot and wore the most fashionable and beautiful outfits I could find. On the inside I was miserable and longed to be smaller size.

As I moved into adulthood it got easier to be overweight. After all, lots of other women were overweight too. I no longer felt like the "only one". I can't say that made it all better – but it did make it more bearable.

Still I longed to be thin. I dreamed about being thin. I planned how I would get thin. I tried every kind of diet. I tried diets that were well balanced and fad diets where I ate only cabbage or only bananas for several days at a time. Every diet brought some good results. Then as soon as the "diet" was over I would put the pounds back on.

I had the standard adult American closet. I had fat clothes, medium clothes and skinny clothes. After every holiday season, I went to the closet to find the "fat clothes". I hated the process but I repeated it year after year. I had more New Year's Resolutions about losing weight. I had more planned and failed diets.

Finally, at age 43 my weight got to an all time high. I wore a size 16. I made every excuse I could make. It was my metabolism. It was my age– it was not exercising enough. As I looked over the last 10 years I could see that with each passing year I was putting on 5 – 10 pounds. I was really frightened by that. I knew if I did nothing and my weight continued to climb I would be in real trouble.

I knew I had to lose the weight. But how? Previously, all of my weight loss plans included the idea of losing weight very quickly. Now, after more than 30 years of trying for quick weight loss I finally had this revelation: What if I just decided to lose it slowly? What if I accepted that there was no "quick fix"?

It was with those thoughts that I embarked on a weight loss journey that would change my life. I finally just accepted that it would not happen quickly. I finally just accepted that while all of my "other diets" produced a 3 – 5 pound weight loss per week it wasn't permanent. Perhaps losing 1 – 2 pounds per week would yield more fruitful and permanent results. I also consulted with my primary care physician to get the clearance on starting a weight loss and workout program. *

*This is a must for anyone that wants to start a weight loss and/or fitness program.

# THE FIRST WEIGH IN
# "BLACK MONDAY"

With that in mind I joined Weight Watchers. I call that first weigh in day "Black Monday". I wanted to cry. I was sure the scale was wrong. I wanted to run from the building screaming and crying. But I told myself, I would stick with this and that nothing would get better unless I really tried.

If your desire is to lose weight the idea of a scale may petrify you. I know it did me. This is the first step. In order to conquer a fear you must face it. It may be difficult but the truth is it's probably bugging you already. So go ahead and face it. This was my first step to conquering my weight problem. I had to face that I weighed more than I have ever in my entire life. I weighed more on what I call "Black Monday" than I weighed when I was nine months pregnant.

Face it and then you can conquer it !!!

## AN OVERVIEW OF THE FIRST FEW WEEKS

The first two months were absolutely awful in terms of making healthy eating changes. First of all I didn't like most of the "healthy food choices". Although there are plenty of healthy foods to pick from I just didn't want to eat them. I wasn't interested in fruits/vegetables/whole grains and correct portion sizes. What did I want? I really wanted a snicker's bar, or nacho cheese Doritos with chip dip. Lots of chip dip.

I don't share this part of my journey to discourage you. I share it to be honest and say whatever your fears or particular challenges are they can be faced and changed. For me I loved junk food and sweets – your issues may be quite different but they can be overcome. What are your issues? Snacking? Sweets? Combo meals? Portion sizes? Too much eating out? Not sure just yet? Try and identify your challenges. Pray about them too.

For me cokes, sweets, and junk food were the problem. For my entire life I just never ate healthy foods on a regular basis. I didn't like vegetables. I didn't eat much fruit. I mostly ate fast food, sugar laden snacks like cookies, Milky Ways, Hershey's with almonds, and of course lots of my favorite beverage Classic Coca Cola. In fact, I drank at least two 20 ounce bottles of Classic Coca Cola a day.

This made the Weight Watchers diet difficult. This would make any healthy diet difficult. How in the world did any one person eat 4 or 5 servings of fruits/vegetables in a day anyway? Perhaps they meant in a year. Certainly they meant in a year. But they didn't mean in a year and there were moments that I thought…..I just can't do this. I'm too old – I've eaten this way for too long. I can't change. I can't lose the weight.

Nonetheless, I decided that I was going to stick with it. I was going to lose the weight this time. I was hungry –absolutely hungry and headachy for the first two months because I couldn't/wouldn't make myself eat healthy foods on a regular basis. Now we all probably know that we can eat plenty of the right foods and still lose weight – the tricky part at this point for me was simply that I didn't like the foods I could select from. Strange as it sounds, I decided to handle this dilemma with prayer.

First, I prayed to lose weight. Then that prayer changed. I began to pray for the courage to change my eating habits. Yes, I felt very strange about praying that prayer. Was it okay for a person to ask God the creator of the universe to help them eat more healthfully? I wondered how spiritual that prayer was – but I prayed it by faith anyway.

In case you're wondering that prayer was not answered instantaneously. Things continued to be difficult. In some ways I was still miserable and hungry for "junk food". But I persisted and did the best I could do. I followed the meal and snack plan. I continued to pray for the courage to change. Gradually things began to get better. After a few weeks I even started to like some of the new foods I was trying.

This same approach to RSYL will work for you. I am glad to share my journey along with its challenges with you. As you pray and seek God to help you make this change (whether it's losing weight or another issue) He will help you. The answer may not be instantaneous and there may be some challenges and distractions. But as you are diligent and persistent you will see results and positive changes.

Think about what changes you want to make as you RSYL. Do you want to develop healthier eating habits and/or start working out? Are you willing to re-work your schedule? Pray about your priorities and daily routine. List the challenges in re-working your schedule below and ask God for wisdom on how to over come those situations.

# WEIGHING IN AND WRITING IT DOWN

List some of the changes you'd like to make as you RSYL. Write down how you might need to re-work your schedule to create more time to work out and/or make healthy food choices.

_____

_____

_____

_____

_____

_____

_____

_____

_____

_____

_____

_____

_____

_____

_____

_____

_____

_____

_____

_____

_____

_____

_____

_____

_____

_____

_____

_____

*Prayer* - Father, I ask you to help me as I embark on this RSYL journey. Give me wisdom in my life and schedule. Bless me with understanding and help me align my priorities with your perfect will. *AMEN*

As you pray about RSYL you will also want to clear what I call the "clutter" from your life and your head. You know all the lies and garbage that sometimes we believe. We might have the belief that once we lose weight all of our problems will be solved. We might believe that people that are thin "have it all together". We might think that if we had more time, more money, better DNA then we wouldn't have to fight this RSYL journey. Your journey will be more successful if you renew your mind in the truth on a daily basis.

### Renew your Mind in the Truth

### Romans 12:2 (NLT)

**Don't copy the behavior and customs of this world, but let God transform you into a new person by changing the way you think. Then you will learn to know God's will for you, which is good and pleasing and perfect.**

This renewing of your mind applies to your thought life. A lot of times we are hanging on to a lot of negative thoughts that are absolutely NOT helping us at all.

Here are some examples of negative worldly thinking:

I'm Fat

I'm Worthless

I can't lose weight

I'm a glutton

It's in my DNA

I can't stop eating

I don't have time

I have to starve to lose weight !!

I have a slow metabolism

Everything I eat goes to my hips……

It's because I'm older

It's because I am a woman

Before you say but it's true I can't stop eating or I don't have time to work out, take a moment and think about how different things might be if you were willing to change how you think? I am asking you to renew your mind in God's truth and not necessarily in the facts and circumstances of your life. Clear that clutter. It's okay to say right now I don't feel like I can stop eating but as you clear the clutter from your thought life that will change. Think on God's Word. Think about how through Jesus you can do all things and that means **all things**.

Replace that clutter with what God says about you. Here are some examples:

### *Psalm 139:14* (New Living Translation)

**Thank you for making me so wonderfully complex!
Your workmanship is marvelous—how well I know it.**

You are wonderfully and fearfully made by the Creator of the Universe. This means you have great value. There is no room for thinking negatively about yourself. God loves you and ascribes great value to your life. He wants your success – He made you wonderfully.

### Romans 8:37 (NLT)

**No, despite all these things, overwhelming victory is ours**

**through Christ, who loved us.**

This means we all have tests and trials. After all, you can't be a conqueror unless you've had a problem or trial. But, He's made you a conqueror. The focus is not on your weight problem or any other problem. The focus when you renew your mind and clear the clutter is how victorious He's made you. How He has given you a conquering overcoming spirit. You can conquer anything as you rely on Him and seek Him.

## Romans 8:11 (NLT)

**The Spirit of God, who raised Jesus from the dead, lives in you. And just as God raised Christ Jesus from the dead, he will give life to your mortal bodies by this same Spirit living within you.**

If you're a believer His Spirit resides in you giving you power to succeed. Quite honestly, this is an advantage the world doesn't have. This means you can RSYL – you can be successful. The Spirit of the Living God resides inside of you quickening you giving you power and energy to succeed. Think on this and it will change your day and change your life. You'll start seeing things in a different light. You'll see things in His light.

## Philippians 4:13 NLT

**"For I can do everything through Christ, who gives me strength."**

This means exactly what it says -- we can do all things through Christ because He is the one giving us strength. He gives us the strength to Right Size our lives as we ask Him and seek Him. Ask Him today to give you the strength you need to Right Size your life and make any changes you need to make.

## Hebrews 13: 6 NLT

**"So we can say with confidence,**

**"The LORD is my helper,
so I will have no fear.
What can mere people do to me?"[**

### *Weighing In Week # 2 ("I only lost 1.6 lbs")* <u>*Total Weight Loss 1.6 lbs.*</u>

As far as stepping on the scales, I weighed in once per week. The first week I lost a whopping 1.6 pounds !!! I was so discouraged I wanted to scream and cry all over again. There I was giving up candy, chips, and Doritos and I only lost 1.6 pounds!!!! My first thought was I probably could have been eating combo meals and drinking cokes. I went through all of that hunger and pain for 1.6 pounds?. You've got to be kidding me !!

Others that were in their first week lost 4 – 5 pounds. I was discouraged and hungry. Truth be told nobody notices a 1.6 pound weight loss. I kept remembering my motto as I got started "I will not quit". This is something as you RSYL you will have to keep in the forefront of your mind – I will not quit. I will not quit. I will not quit. You have to be prayerful and determined.

If you have a disappointing week in terms of weight loss or you go off track, refer back to the Clearing the Clutter Section. Begin praying and reciting those verses. Find some other encouraging verses in scripture. Even King David had to encourage himself in the Lord. This is a part of the RSYL journey. Making and maintaining lasting change may have its challenges and ups and downs but you can do it.

### *Weighing In Week # 3 (-4.4lbs)*      <u>*Total Weight Loss 6 lbs.*</u>

I continued on eating healthfully. The next weigh in proved more beneficial. I lost 4.4 pounds. That brought a smile to my face. Finally, some encouragement – some payback for all of my hard work. I even felt like my clothes fit just a little bit looser. That was a good feeling.

When I got the craving for a candy bar – or combo meal I would close my eyes and think about how wonderful it was that my clothes were feeling looser and fitting better. I would close my eyes and think about how much better it felt to be getting smaller and how a combo meal and/or candy would really mess everything up. I would remind myself of how happy I would be in the next smaller size if I could just continue on and forego that combo meal – or candy. The experts call these techniques visualization and anchoring. Regardless of the techniques formal names they were working.

These techniques will work for you too as you RSYL. It will take consistent prayer, determination, and reminders of how much better success feels than eating combo meals/junk food or whatever it is that you enjoy. The RSYL journey is about making lifestyle changes and progressing slowly over time. You will see the results you want as you continue doing the right things. You can RSYL.

Week after week for the first two months I slowly but consistently lost weight. I didn't seem to get the huge losses that others did. My average loss per week was about 1.5 pounds. They say slow and steady wins the race but when you're 43 years old and wearing a size 16 you want things to go more quickly.

After all, I wasn't cheating on the diet plan. I gave up cookies, ice cream, and chips and the weight loss thing stayed slow and steady. I continued to remind myself though that I was losing weight. Yes, it was slow but it was coming off. My clothes were getting too big. There wasn't a struggle each morning anymore as I stood before the closet trying to figure out what wouldn't be too tight – or what would look best. It was getting easier to select outfits and that felt good.

As you RSYL your progress may be slower than you'd like. You've probably watched enough weight loss shows that celebrate the 10 and 15 pound weight losses in just one week. I thank God for all that. It's exciting. In weight loss though slow and steady does win the race. Encourage yourself in the process. Even if it's just 1 or 2 pounds in week it's a loss. Over time a 1 - 2 pound weight loss begins to add up and make a dramatic difference.

*Weighing In Week # 4 (-1.4 lbs)*          *Total Weight Loss 7.4 pounds*

Just one month into the process I was progressing slowly. This is a critical point for most people trying to lose weight. Once you've done something for about a month or so it can be easy to lose the excitement and enthusiasm you had at first. Don't let that happen. Remind yourself of all your successes thus far. Remind yourself of your hard work and how you have progressed. You don't want to turn back now!!!

There is also over the course of a 4 week period ample opportunity for distraction. What I mean by that is by this time certainly someone has invited you out for dinner. Someone has had a holiday or special birthday occasion or something like that. The wonderful thing about RSYL is that none of these events have to throw you off track or deter you from your course.

It's a matter really of understanding that special occasions and events are just a part of life. They are meant to be enjoyed and celebrated and you can do that while losing weight. I've mentioned before that I elected to join Weight Watchers. There are many fine well balanced weight loss programs available. I personally recommend and like Weight Watchers because the plan offers so many options. Again, let me make this clear. I am not employed by Weight Watchers I do not own stock in their company. Personally, I just love their program.

They have great options for eating out. They have pre-packaged foods and dessert options that give you their calorie and point value. For me it worked when going to a celebration to take one of the weight watcher desserts with me. I would eat that at the birthday party or get together. They taste great and allow you to join in the celebration without the risk of going off your food plan.

What's important for you is that you select a food plan that works for you. Select a plan formulated by a nutritionist or a plan that your physician recommends to you. Follow that plan faithfully. Record in a food journal what you eat every single day. You'll be surprised sometimes that you're eating more than what you think. It's important as you RSYL to enlist expert help. I can help you by sharing my story. My RSYL story is offered as practical help from someone who has 'been there". From someone who has lost 70 pounds and kept it off without a problem for 3 years.

Why do you need expert help? Let's face it – if you could do it or if I could have done it on my own we would have done so long ago. We all get to where we are due to our own level of thinking and knowledge. It's critical to consult with people who know more than us. It takes consulting with experts and people who have really been there and have successfully taken the weight off.

Even the Bible says there is wisdom in consulting with others. We are in fact promised success as we consult with the wise about our plans.

### *Proverbs 15:22* NLT

**Plans go wrong for lack of advice;
many advisers bring success.**

So as you embark on the RSYL journey enlist expert help. People are usually far more willing to help than we imagine. It's critical to have a support and buddy system to ensure long term success. It helps us keep the enthusiasm and momentum to have others along with us.

Journaling is an excellent way to keep yourself on track. Every month there will be an opportunity to record in RSYL how you're doing. You'll find this invaluable in terms of recording and meeting your goals.

# WEIGHING IN AND WRITING IT DOWN

Record this month's weight loss and fitness goals, your progress, and challenges. Next to each challenge write down how you plan to overcome that challenge.

Have you been praying about how to RSYL - record your specific prayers and answers below:

_____

_____

_____

_____

_____

_____

_____

_____

_____

_____

_____

_____

_____

_____

_____

_____

_____

_____

_____

_____

_____

_____

_____

_____

_____

_____

_____

_____

_____

---

*Prayer* - Father, I ask right now in Jesus Name that you'll give me the strength to continue Right Sizing my Life. I ask you Father by the power of your Holy Spirit to help me renew my mind in what you say about me. I ask you Father to put good people in my life that can help mentor me on this journey. Thank you for giving me the strength to embark on this journey. Crown my efforts with success. ***AMEN***

### *Weighing In Week # 5* (-1 lb)          *Total Weight Loss of 8.4 lbs.*

At this point I can start to tell a difference. A real difference. Now I am excited about the progress. It no longer seems so slow. Well perhaps its still seems slow but I recognize the payoff. This is critical to your RSYL journey. Recognize the payoff. Don't look at all that you're giving up. Look at what you're getting rid of – you are getting rid of excess weight. You are getting rid of excuses. You are getting rid of obstacles and challenges.

You are facing your life and taking dominion. That's what God wants for you. That's what God wants for me. He wants for us to walk in dominion in a godly confidence of who we are. Right now you are beginning to see the correlation between food choices, portion sizes, consistency and weight loss results. This correlation will continue to be important to you throughout the journey and then also as you maintain your goal weight. Yes, if you are faithful to this process you will reach your goal weight and you will be able to maintain it.

### *Weighing In Week # 6* (-1 lb.)          *Total Weight Loss of 9.4 lbs.*

I so wanted to have a total weight loss of 10 pounds this week. I had to settle for 9.4 lbs. I figured I was close. That's important to this process. Set goals. Set moderate goals. Give yourself some slack though also. The important thing is to eat right consistently and the weight loss will happen over time.

### *Weighing In Week #7* (- 2.0 lbs)     <u>*Total Weight Loss of 11.4 lbs.*</u>

Obviously, this was a good week for me. Every week will vary. It's important to understand this. You won't hit the same numbers each week. Sometimes it will be more sometimes it may be less.

At this time I start considering working out. Remember I had never in my entire life worked out regularly. I had tried it on occasion but never consistently. I did consult with my physician (which is a must for you too). You must have medical clearance before embarking on any weight loss or workout program. You want to make sure it's safe for you to diet and exercise. My physician gave me the go ahead.

I started thinking about, researching and also praying about what workout regime I might start. You might want to do the same thing. You need clearance from your doctor but then you also need wisdom in selecting a workout program. Pick something that you like. If you don't like it you'll never stick with. Do some research about fitness programs. Take your time and select what you feel you're most likely to stick with.

It took me several more weeks to start working out. Remember I was praying and working up the courage. I was afraid to start working out. I was afraid I couldn't do it. I was afraid to go to a fitness center. You may not have these same fears. In fact, I hope you don't. If you do though you can work and pray through them. God really does delight in the details of our lives. As we do our part He does His.

*"All our dreams can come true - if we have the courage to pursue them."*
~Walt Disney

### *Weighing In Week # 8* (- .6 lbs)     <u>*Total Weight Loss 12 lbs.*</u>

I'm now 2 months into the process. This is getting to be more of a routine for me. In fact, it's truly getting easier in many ways. Pre-planning what I am going to eat is becoming easier. Recording every meal and snack in the food journal is just a part of the RSYL process now. These things are starting to be a habit. It's no longer feeling like "extra" work. It's just part of living. I see the results these new habits are bringing. I like the results. This is much better than feeling overweight and worrying about what size I wear. Certainly, its work but its work well invested.

I'm still thinking about working out. I haven't made any firm decisions. You may have already started working out. If you have – good for you. If you're still on the sidelines thinking about it (like me) then keep thinking, praying and planning. You'll get that in motion soon I am sure.

When you are at the two month point you will really see some the benefits of your new lifestyle. The new habits are becoming second nature. That's what we want. The new habits to become a new lifestyle. A healthier more positive lifestyle.

> *"Wise words bring many benefits*
>
> *and hard work brings rewards."*
>
> **Proverbs 12:14 NLT**

# WEIGHING IN AND WRITING IT DOWN

Have you started to work out yet? If so, record what you're doing. If you're still thinking about working out take some time to list your options and weigh the pros and cons. Also, are you keeping a daily food journal? Are you writing down everything you eat? Are you reviewing the journal to see where you're doing well and where you might need some improvement/s? Record this months weight loss and fitness goals, your progress, and challenges.

_____

_____

_____

_____

_____

_____

_____

_____

_____

_____

_____

_____

_____

_____

_____

_____

_____

_____

_____

_____

_____

_____

_____

_____

_____

_____

_____

***Prayer*** - Father, help me to begin working out and take care of the temple that you have given me. Give the courage to be consistent. Help me find the time to work out and stick with it. God, open up my eyes to all of the opportunities you have placed before me. Make this journey fun and interesting and help me see Father how you delight in the details of my life. ***AMEN***

# OVERVIEW OF MONTHS 2 & 3

I reach an important goal.

I experience a miracle in the Kroger produce department.

I start to work out.

### *Weighing In Week # 9* (-.4 lbs)        *Total Weight Loss 12.4 lbs*

Well, I had lost a total of 12.4 lbs.  I had a speaking engagement coming up and I was grateful for that weight loss.  At this point I set a goal for myself that by the speaking engagement I would be able to fit into a beautiful purple suit that had hung in my closet for 3 years (tags still on it) but had never been able to wear.  Do you have any clothes like that?  Clothes you just can't throw away because you just might be able to wear them someday?  I know how that feels and I so understand.  Perhaps as you RSYL you can set some goals to get back into those outfits.  Just set reasonable, attainable goals.  That helps set the stage for success.

Whenever I was tempted to go off the food plan for any reason I would close my eyes, pray, and think about how wonderful it would be to actually fit into that purple suit.  Just that small amount of time in prayer and focusing on the goal gave me the power to overcome the food temptation.

Use this process in your RSYL journey.  Whether your goal is an actual weight loss amount, work out goal or wearing a smaller size put the goal before you daily.  Think on it.  Pray on it.  Work toward it.

I began to see how God truly gives us strength in every single area of our lives.

### *Weighing In Week # 10* (- 2.2 lbs)    *Total Weight Loss 14.6 lbs*

The total weight loss is almost at 15 pounds. I decide to go ahead and just call it 15 pounds even !! At this point, I begin to really believe that I can stick this out for the long-haul. Every single day I take time to pray and clear the clutter from my thought life. I ask God to give me courage. I ask God for strength and He does. Not always perhaps in the ways I like but He helped me. His help did not mean that I never felt hungry. His help did not mean that the way was easy. But He did make a way.

I continue weighing in only once per week. Please don't weigh more than once per week. It can be discouraging. We all have normal fluctuations with our weight that are not the result of gaining fat. Pretty much the experts say weigh once per week on the same day, about the same time and the same scale. This will give you the most accurate measure of your weight loss.

Along with weekly weigh-ins I visit my closet for clothes that were previously too small. I found it very motivational to fit into things (or at least get closer) that I couldn't wear previously. These were just some visual reminders that weight loss was happening. Actually, I found this part more enjoyable than the weekly weigh-ins.

It's important to be able to reinforce our success. If trying on clothes that were previously too small is an encouragement to you do that. Reviewing your food journal will help you see you progress and determination. Just anything that is meaningful to you.

Continue also to pray and meditate on scripture. Keep your thought life renewed. You are making some major changes and you need His help to make those changes and to make those changes last.

**Weighing In Week # 11** (-1.0 lbs)      ***Total Weight Loss 15.6 lbs***

I had never lasted on a diet or eating plan for this long. I had always given up prior to this point previously. In some ways I am amazed that I am hanging in there. I believe having a Weight Watcher buddy helps me. I know she plans on going to each meeting with me so it helps keep me accountable. Her positive attitude and approach also encourages me. My weight watcher buddy was excited with any loss. Her smile and enthusiasm cheered me up on those days when my weight loss was very small.

Hopefully, you've got someone in the process with you. If not, you can still achieve success. You'll have to keep focused on encouraging yourself. The truth is that even though it's helpful to have someone in the process with you, it is when it's all said and done an individual choice. It is a choice that you can make and achieve results.

It's almost speaking engagement time. I've been looking and re-looking at the beautiful purple suit. Will it fit? Will I reach that goal? Only time will tell.

**Weighing In Week # 12** (-1.0 lbs)      ***Total Weight Loss 16.6 lbs***

It's time to find out if the purple suit fits. It's speaking engagement time. My message is ready. I am excited and I am wondering. Did I lose enough weight?

The answer is yes, I did. The suit fit. I was happy and surprised. I mean I thought it would fit but I needed to know for sure. I cannot tell you how elated I was to reach my first concrete goal. I did it !!!

It was wonderful for me to be able to put on the purple suit for that speaking engagement. It fit – it actually fit. It was at this point that I realized on a new level that the struggle of changing was worth it. Resisting combo meals – candy – chips was actually beginning to work. My time in prayer about the courage to change my eating habits was starting to pay off too.

At the beginning of the diet I was so hungry and had lots of headaches. While there were a plethora of good food choices available to me – I just didn't want those healthy foods. Instead I hungered for fat soaked foods. Then one day (it seemed out of the blue) while I was grocery shopping I noticed that I actually liked being in the produce department.

Now if you knew me at all you would know how funny that really is. I mean I'm the woman who just one-year prior had to ask someone what cabbage looked like while I was in the produce section. The woman I asked politely helped me and then asked me, "Aren't you the woman on Christian television?" I said yes though meekly and introduced myself.

Boy was I embarrassed. I was a grown woman and I had hosted a daily television show for almost 9 years and I had no idea what cabbage looked like. That was the truth. I just didn't eat vegetables growing up and as an adult I didn't have any real plans to change until I realized that I was growing larger each and every year and that I wasn't comfortable with the weight gain or having to buy larger clothing each and every year.

Let's go back to enjoying the produce department. I remembered how I had been praying for the courage to change my eating habits. I had been praying that for about 3 months and now "seemingly out of the blue" the produce section looks good. I mean I bought spinach, carrots, mushrooms, and assorted other vegetables.

Funny as it may sound these were items I never ate before. I went home and ate a spinach salad (no dressing). I absolutely loved it. No kidding. Literally, praying for the courage to change – changed my thinking and my taste buds. I promise you that never before in my life did I even consider eating vegetables. Now here I was eating a spinach salad. I loved the spinach salad. It was good.

It may sound very strange but I learned truly firsthand how God helps us make change. It may not happen in a moment or a day but over time as we are persistent we will see God answer.

The answered prayer was pivotal for me. I was able to eat more simply because I like vegetables now. The truth is we can have a good amount of food if it's healthy. God never intended for us to starve He wants us to be nourished and to enjoy healthy food. It's part of the abundant life.

*Weighing In Week # 13* (-1.0 lbs)      *Total Weight Loss 17.6 lbs.*

# STARTING TO WORK OUT

Well if healthful eating was foreign to me – working out was even stranger concept. It's not that I didn't know anything about working out – after all I had been a card-carrying member of Sports Village a fitness center for years. It's just that I never used that membership. I was just paying the membership fee but not receiving any of the benefits.

Just as I was making plans to use that membership I noticed an ad in the paper for the "Next Biggest Loser". The ad for Next Biggest Loser was from Sports Village where I was already a card-carrying member. When I called to get more information I learned that it was basically a weight loss and work out program with a team concept. Each team had a specific trainer and worked out together three times per week. I was absolutely petrified but I decided to "give it a try".

After all, the team concept really appealed to me. Previously, I never felt comfortable in a workout facility but being a part of a team made me feel more at ease. Barry was our team trainer and he had lost over 100 pounds and kept it off successfully. That provided him instant credibility with me. I also felt comfortable with him knowing that he understood my concerns since he had traveled this journey himself.

The team concept helped me in a lot of ways. First of all, it helped me to see that others were in the same situation as me. It was similar to the "buddy concept" and had built in accountability for each team member.

I can still remember how difficult that first Next Biggest Loser meeting was for me. I was so nervous. I didn't like the weigh–in and the measuring. Now I had to weigh in 2 times per week. Once at Weight Watchers and once at the Sports Village. Even though I was a few pounds lighter I still didn't like weigh-ins. I was still convinced that there was something wrong with the scales!!! I tried standing on them more "lightly" but the results were always the same. This working out was a whole new venture for me. I was intimidated and yet excited. I knew I had to take this new step by faith.

The first few work-outs seemed awful too. I couldn't keep up. I mean half the time I wasn't even sure I understood the instructions – or the point of what we were trying to do. They would say "hold your abs in" and I would think, seriously?

The workouts were a combination of cardio and weight training. It didn't matter the combination though – I just didn't like it. I mean who likes anything that's really hard and makes you feel like you're just not adequate? I felt about as ungraceful as you can get and the movements seemed so unnatural.

Nevertheless, I stayed faithful and consistent. I showed up each meeting and sure enough it got easier each time. Now I won't go so far as to say that working out was enjoyable yet – but it was a new habit in the making.

For me, working out with a trainer made all of the difference. First of all, even though we worked out in teams – I still got some individual attention. This was of immense help because I really knew nothing about working out. Secondly, the trainer, Barry, was very encouraging and patient. He truly had our best interests at heart. Should you decide to work out with a trainer select someone that you feel comfortable with. It's important for you to feel comfortable. You need to be able to ask questions. Select someone that you can talk to and share your goals and fears. It may take a little research and some time to find a trainer that's right for you. It's no different than finding the right hair stylist – doctor – or counselor.  Keep looking until you find a trainer that's right for you.

# ALL OR NOTHING WORKOUTS

In the past when I tried working out it was definitely the "all or nothing" concept. What usually ended up happening was I would get way too sore – hurt myself – or just plain burn out. Then, I would just QUIT working out.

I remember one time that I specifically set out to make up for lost time. Yes, I started working out with a vengeance. I gave it everything I had. I gave 110%. On the fourth day I woke up so sore I could barely walk. I ended up having to use a sports cream for muscle soreness that had a very strong and unpleasant odor. Yes, that's right you could smell me at least a block away. It was embarrassing and I was really hurting. This is exactly the kind of thing you want to avoid as you step out to RSYL.

Having a trainer helped me apply the slow and steady philosophy into my workout. The key is to work out hard enough that it's a challenge but not so hard that you can't walk or do regular everyday activity. Sure there will be some muscle soreness. But it should be at a manageable level. A trainer can help you with this because this is their area of expertise. Sure enough each week I would see some progress. Each week I would lose weight and could work out a little harder. Once I started seeing consistent progress it was easier to make working out a priority in my life.

Nonetheless, along the way there were many reasons to quit. I developed tendonitis at one point; - I got an upper respiratory infection a few weeks later and had to miss some classes. Additionally, there were periods of time where my work schedule would get really busy. My family life also got hectic. Pretty much there was always something presenting itself to me as a reason to give up and or give in. Don't be deterred by disruptions in schedule. Get back on track.

I truly believe that having the trainer and the team concept was a major reason I continued to go back after each "setback". I felt like there were people depending on me to help the team - and my trainer had done so much to help me so I wanted to stick with it. Develop some sort of buddy system of accountability method to ensure your success.

Also, whenever I felt like I just wanted to skip the work out and go home I would remind myself of how lousy I would feel later. I would remind myself how I never regretted working out once the work out was done. But I always regretted when I missed a work out. This is just a part of developing discipline. Discipline is an essential quality in business, family, and just life in general. Successful people are disciplined. If you want to be successful in RSYL this means you must develop discipline. It won't be easy but you can do it.

After adding workouts to my weight loss plan I began to see the whole picture come into play. In fact, I began to see a lot of differences. The weight loss picked up just a little bit and the physical changes were apparent. Now my clothes were really getting too big. People were starting to notice. More importantly I could see the differences and that meant everything to me.

*Better to be patient than powerful; better to have self-control than to conquer a city.*

*Proverbs 6:21 NLT*

# WEIGHING IN AND WRITING IT DOWN

Are you familiar with the all or nothing workouts - or even the all or nothing eating plans? Are you settled on the slow and steady approach? This is an opportunity to write what you've been thinking about and what decisions you've made in terms of your weight loss and fitness plans. Record this months weight loss and fitness goals, your progress, and challenges. Next to each challenge write down how you plan to overcome that challenge.

_____
_____
_____
_____
_____
_____
_____
_____
_____
_____
_____
_____
_____
_____
_____
_____
_____
_____
_____
_____
_____
_____
_____
_____
_____
_____

***Prayer*** Father thank you that I even have the desire to Right Size My Life. Now give me the determination and dedication it takes to make these changes. Help me have the desire to workout and lead me to the plan that will be best for me physically and will also work for my time schedule. Thank you Father that Nothing is impossible for me because I believe and put my trust in you. ***AMEN.***

# OVERVIEW OF MONTHS 4 & 5

The "Slow and Steady Approach" for lasting results

Right Sizing your portions

Hitting the dreaded "plateau"

Dealing with Naysayers, Doubters, & Sabotage

*Weighing In Week # 14 - 4.4* **lbs**          *Total Weight Loss 22 lbs.*

## SLOW AND STEADY WINS
## THE WEIGHT-LOSS RACE

Most people attempting to lose weight want to do so as quickly as possible. Of course we've all heard people say "you didn't put it on in a day and you won't lose it in a day either". Those were always such discouraging words to me. They were true but not comforting, unless you really learn to understand and embrace the weight loss process.

According to Mayo Clinic physical medicine and rehabilitation specialist Edward Laskowski, M.D. fast weight loss is usually followed by rapid weight gain. Besides 1 pound of fat contains 3,500 calories so you need to burn 500 more calories than you eat each day just to lose 1 pound per week. If you're losing more than 1 – 2 pounds per week, it's either water weight or lean tissue you're losing, not fat. Weight loss of 1-2 pounds per week may seem like an agonizingly slow pace but if improving your health is a long-term goal the speed of your weight loss isn't important.

I remind myself that slow and steady is key to improving your health and keeping the weight off forever. I also remind myself also that I must shed the "lose weight quickly" mentality in order to achieve my goals. Research and experts concur that people who lose weight slowly are more successful in keeping the weight off. So if you're tired and losing and gaining embrace the concept of losing weight slowly and steadily and then you'll be more likely to keep that weight off forever.

### Over Half of Adults in America are overweight

As you are on the RSYL journey it can be easy to feel like you're all alone. It can seem that you are the only one working hard to lose weight or that there are lots of people who are just "naturally thin" or unconcerned about their weight. Actually, statistics also show that a majority of Americans are struggling with weight issues. This fact alone, should encourage us to make the changes we need to make and Right size our lives.

Look at the breakdown below provided by the American Sports Data, the National Center for Health Statistics, and the Society for Women's Health Research and the Centers for Disease Control and Prevention

| Vital Stats | Men | Women |
|---|---|---|
| Average Weight | 198.4 lbs | 164.7 lbs |
| Percentage who are overweight | 67.2% | 61.9% |
| Percentage who are obese | 27.5% | 33.4% |
| Percentage trying to lose weight | 28.8% | 43.6% |

*Statistics from American Sports Data, the National Center for Health Statistics, The Society for Women's Health Research and the Centers for Disease Control and Prevention.

The fact is you are not alone, over half the American adult population is overweight. In a sense it can be helpful to know that overweight is an issue that affects over half the adult population in America. It gives us insight in terms of how our culture may play a role in our fight against obesity and excess weight. The overweight problem of course in its most raw form is consuming more calories than we burn. When you consider though the standard American fare – fast food – fat laden foods – extra large portions it only stands to reason that over half the adult American population is overweight. I say this to point out that it's not really in most cases our DNA – nor is it necessarily gluttony – or gender necessarily. It's our culture and lifestyle. Understanding this issue can help us take responsibility, make prayerful changes and get rid of undue guilt, worry, and blame.

### *Weighing In Week # 15* (- .6 lbs)     *Total Weight Loss 22.6 lbs.*

## OUR EYES ARE BIGGER THAN OUR STOMACHS – A LESSON IN PORTION SIZES

One of the things that I find really helpful in my RSYL journey is learning about portion sizes. Now I have to tell you I didn't really care for the term "portion sizes." I couldn't believe that a chicken breast was supposed to be the size of a deck of cards – or computer mouse. I mean tell me that last time that you went to a restaurant and were served a chicken breast the size of a computer mouse or deck of cards. Truth be told most restaurant portions are at least double the correct portion size.

It's no wonder over half of America is struggling with being overweight. Portion sizes are growing by leaps and bounds. Now, a portion simply defined is a helping of food. Think about all those recipes you've made over the years. Ever thought about how it says the recipe should feed six but when you put it on your dinner table it feeds four? Or how about your favorite package of chips? When you look at the nutrition label you see that a serving is 150 calories. Then you think that's not so bad. When you read the nutrition label more closely you see that a serving (or portion) actually consists of 5 whole chips. Who eats just 5 chips?

Our eyes really are bigger than our stomachs and we've come to accept as normal larger portion sizes. In fact, this kind of supersized thinking is everywhere. Television, radio, and print advertising. We've been conditioned to think that bigger is better and it shows on every level. Even beverages these days are huge. The truth is there is no way for the average person to eat all that food and maintain a normal healthy weight.

Part of RSYL is to develop a new pattern of thinking about portion sizes. Once your thinking is renewed this process will become easier for you. I know you're probably thinking but I need all that food. That's what it takes to fill me up. But the truth is our stomach is only the size of about an average fist and we don't need all that food. We've just been conditioned to think that we do.

### Portion Size Examples

3 Ounces Protein = Size of a deck of cards

Banana = Size of a cell phone

Potato = Size of a light bulb

Apple= Size of Tennis Ball

Green Salad = A Baseball or fist

Visit the website below for a comprehensive list of examples and visuals on correct portion sizes.

http://www.webmd.com/diet/healthtool-portion-size-plate

Get these portion sizes in your head. When you look at your plate before you take a bite figure out what you can actually eat. Just look at your plate and when you see a huge chicken breast on the plate visualize the deck of cards and just eat that portion. That goes for everything on your plate. Visualize your portion sizes first. Commit to what amount you will and won't eat. This may be hard at first but it's like any habit the more you do it the easier it will get. Very shortly, this habit will become automatic for you. You will no longer have to think or struggle you will just know how to visualize your plate and eat accordingly.

When you look at your actual plate make sure it's not oversized. This will undermine the process. Use a regular sized plate not a serving platter disguised as a plate. Most plates at restaurants are way too large. They are in many instances serving platters. When one of those platters is placed in front of you visualize a normal sized plate. Practicing correct portion sizing and dividing up your plate are skills that can be learned and will take you through any situation without throwing you off your course.

### *"If it tastes too good – you should probably spit it out".*

Bobbi Mofield, Personal Trainer Extraordinaire

Part of RSYL is learning how to think properly about food. It's understanding that knowledge is power. That knowing the right amount to eat is essential to your current and long term success. As you develop this skill you will grow in confidence. You will no longer fear going out with friends to restaurants because it will throw you off your "diet". By RSYL, you will learn how to go anywhere and everywhere and stay on course. This is the whole idea of enjoying the life that God gave us. You can go out to eat – go to parties and participate in regular real life activities while you are losing weight and once you're in the maintenance phase.

### *"Never, I mean never clean your plate."*

Barry Campbell, Personal Trainer

### *Weighing In Week # 16* (- .8 lbs)    <u>*Total Weight Loss 23.4 lbs.*</u>

Wow, I lost a whole 1.4 pounds in two weeks. Talk about slow. What happened did I hit a plateau? As I've shared I'm not an expert in diet and fitness. Rather, I'm an ordinary person that embarked upon a journey to Right Size my Life. When you talk about a 1.4 pound weight loss in two weeks I believe we could call that a plateau. A plateau is a period or phase in which there is little increase or decrease. For me, it was very little decrease.

Lots of dieters say they experience plateaus. I did. I can tell you it's frustrating. Especially because I was seriously following my weight loss plan and workout regimen. I wasn't "cheating". I was consistent in my work-outs and yet the scale recorded little change.

What should you do if as you are RSYL and you hit a plateau? The experts have a lot of suggestions and I'll share some of those in just a little bit. Here's what I did:

I stayed faithful in my food plan and with my food journal.

I increased the cardio in my workouts by 30 minutes 3 x per week

I encouraged myself that plateaus are a normal and necessary part of the journey. I refused to dwell on the negative. I also did not listen to any of the following comments offered by well intentioned people:

### *"The closer you get to your goal the harder it is to lose"*

I understand that you are thinking but Monica that's true. So what? So what if it's true. Just hang in there. Keep at it. You will push through the plateau. Don't worry about how hard it is. Think about some of the challenges you've already faced and taken steps to address.

Making the decision to lose weight.

Deciding to live a healthier lifestyle.

Finding the energy to change your daily routine.

Every one of these things shows that you are not afraid to face the "tough stuff". You can face a plateau. A plateau is easy compared to some of the other things in life you've faced. Just stick with your food plan and increase your cardio. You will break through this plateau with persistence and determination.

### *"You might be at your set point"*

Again the experts have a lot to say about set points. Here's the proper question to ask yourself. Are you at your goal weight? Have you discussed this goal weight with your physician or other expert that's helping you? If you have set a reasonable goal (within the BMI charts) and you are not at goal weight yet then you are probably not at your set point but rather you are at a plateau. You can break through a plateau. You've faced much tougher things in your life. You can face this in victory too.

One of the most essential tools during a plateau is a food journal. In fact, a food journal is critical for the entire journey. A food journal makes us accountable with how much we're eating. The experts report that we eat more food than we think we eat. This means that we are usually taking in more calories than we think we are. Review your food journal carefully. Make sure you haven't changed or added anything. If you've changed something go back to what you were doing. If you haven't changed anything hang in there and remember as you consistently do the right things you will reap the right results. It may take some time and you may hit a plateau here or there but you will breakthrough.

### *Weighing In Week # 17* (-1.5 lbs)     *Total Weight Loss 24.9 lbs.*

Okay I feel like I broke through the plateau. That's good. That's really good. Most of the feedback I get from others is positive and encouraging. Now though that I am making some progress and that the results are getting more visible I start hearing some other comments as well.

These comments I refer to as "negative". They may not always seem negative some may actually be framed as a compliment. But they have the power to deter you from your course if you don't understand what's happening. Here are some examples of "negative" comments that come from naysayers and doubters. Ever heard of any of these comments?

**"You don't need to lose any more weight"**

**"One bite won't make you fat."**

**"This little bit won't hurt you."**

**"Working out will make you hungrier"**

**(If you're a woman they will say) "working out will make you too muscular"**

**"You're too old to lose weight."**

**"It's your metabolism"**

**"It's in your DNA"**

If you want to RSYL you can't listen to these types of comments. These kinds of comments are myths, fables, and sometimes just plain old jealousy. Sometimes the green eyed monster gets even the best of people. Avoid meditating on these types of statements. Remind yourself how important it is for you to RSYL. Remind yourself of all the benefits – what you have to gain by staying faithful to the path.

In fact, at this point it may be good for you to make a list about why you want to RSYL. After you written down the reasons why you want to RSYL make a plan and how you will do it. It can be as simple as:

**Sample list on why I want to Right Size**

1. I want to be healthier.

2. I want to wear a smaller size.

3. I want to get to goal weight before the family reunion (or whatever the event is)

**Practical Steps on how I will Right Size**

1. I will follow a reasonable well balanced eating plan (for me it was Weight Watchers)

2. I will workout 3 times per week consistently. (Run walk, ride a bike, take a class just do something and be consistent).

3. I will practice Right Sizing my plate by learning proper portion sizes.

# WEIGHING IN AND WRITING IT DOWN

Take this opportunity to write down why you want to RSYL. List the practical steps you will take to achieve your goals. This include your goals to Right Size portions and work-out consistently. You may need to think about what you need to change in your schedule. What can you give up or cut out to make the appropriate time to work out?

_____

_____

_____

_____

_____

_____

_____

_____

_____

_____

_____

_____

_____

_____

_____

_____

_____

_____

_____

_____

_____

_____

_____

_____

_____

_____

_____

*Prayer* - Father, give me wisdom and discipline to Right size my portions. Help me also Father to evaluate my schedule. Show me how to steward my life so that I can take care of my temple. Help me to see things from your perspective. ***AMEN***

*Weighing In Week # 18* (- **2.0 lbs**)     *Total Weight Loss 26.9 lbs.*

One of the things that I learned on my RSYL journey is that nothing absolutely nothing can replace persistence, consistency and diligence. That's right there are diets that promise you can lose 30 pounds in 30 days. You may have to settle for eating only bananas for 30 days in order to do that but ….what fun – or not!!! Or perhaps a promise to drop 2 dress sizes in 10 days. Whatever, whatever, whatever. That's all fad stuff. Those plans don't usually work for the long term. If they did then almost nobody on the planet would be dieting. Everyone would already be at goal weight.

What works for the long term are the basics. The basics include: persistence, consistency and diligence.

*Persistence*     Continuing…..in spite of opposition, obstacles, discouragement

**Consistency** Constantly adhering to the same principles, course

*Diligence*     constant and earnest effort to accomplish what is undertaken; persistent exertion of body or mind.

> ***"We can do anything we want if we stick to it long enough."***
>
> Helen Keller

One of the things I learned in my journey was the power of persistence, consistency, and diligence. Sometimes, it's not the huge immense effort but the small, consistent steps that make the difference over the long-haul.

Consider for a moment how many diets or work out plans you've tried so far. Think about all the time, money, and effort you've expended with no lasting results. By the time I decided to Right Size My Life I had tried at least 50 diets unsuccessfully. I had paid thousands of dollars over the years on various work out equipment, health club memberships and the like. Clearly, I had expended time, money and effort. My approach however, was what I call the "All or Nothing Syndome".

The "All or Nothing Syndrome" demands a whole lot. In fact, it demands radical eating plans and extreme workouts. Certainly, you'll get some quick results. The question you need to ask yourself though is "do those results last?". If they do then stick with it. If the results don't last then it's time to try something new.

The challenge with the "All or Nothing Syndrome" is that you usually wear out. I mean who can really eat 500 calories per day over the long haul? You know this kind of eating makes you feel deprived and before you know it you're on some kind of binge eating a whole bag of cookies or a large pizza. If you haven't worked out in years or months how are you going to start working out every single day and not wear yourself out?

Now is the time to do things differently and RSYL. One of the greatest tools you have at your disposal (and it costs nothing) is the power of consistency. Slow and steady will win this race.

Granted my journey did not include weigh ins with huge losses. Never in the one year period did I lose 5 pounds in one week. Not even in the first week. But what I did do was lose weight slowly and keep it off. That's what you want. You want to RSYL and then keep it that way – forever. Literally, it has not been a problem for me to keep the weight off. I don't even think about it anymore. Over time I learned new eating habits and started working out. This process went slowly but it became automatic for me. That's just what you want.

***Weighing In Week # 19*** (- **2.0 lbs**)     ***Total Weight Loss 28.9 lbs.***

This is the longest I have ever stuck with a diet. In fact, I'm a little surprised at myself. At the same time I am afraid I will mess up.

It's important as you RSYL to face your fears. By that I don't mean that you should think about your fears all of the time. That would not be good for you at all. Acknowledging your fears though is necessary to overcoming them.

With that in mind acknowledge your fears. Ask God to give you strength to finish what you start. Rehearse your successes. Encourage yourself. Remind yourself of every time you passed on cookies and cake. Think about the times where it could have been easier to go home after a long day's work but you went ahead and worked out anyway. Even King David had to encourage himself and you will have to along the way also.

As you rehearse your successes you will change your thought patterns. It may not happen immediately but over time you will find yourself thinking differently. Don't expect this entire journey to be easy. If it was easy you would have done it by now. It's hard work but it's rewarding. Stick with it. Now is no time to give up.

***Weighing In Week # 20*** (-**1.0 lbs**)     ***Total Weight Loss 29.9 lbs.***

For me, encouraging myself included reviewing my weight loss successes. I would review my weekly weigh in book. I would remind myself how much weight I had lost. As I reviewed each entry I thought about the effort and cost it took and then I congratulated myself on sticking with it.

I would think about the 20 long weeks that it took to lose 29.9 pounds. As I thought about the effort I put forth in that 20 weeks I would see clearly how I had worked too hard to give up now.

Review your weight loss successes often. Success breeds success. This is not bragging or unspiritual. This is a part of encouraging yourself and renewing your mind.

Review your successes. Renew your mind. Train your mind to think positively. This is a godly principle. Your thoughts are powerful

### *Weighing In Week # 21* (- 2.0 lbs)     *Total Weight Loss 31.9 lbs.*

I'm excited that my weigh–in revealed a total loss of 31.9 pounds. I mean really excited. The results are more than making up for the sacrifices. I've been sore from working out almost every day for the last four weeks. I'm tired too. When people ask me if I have more energy now I have to laugh. Not just yet I say. Right now, I'm just sore and tired but I am losing weight.

That's important for you to keep in mind. Everything in the RSYL process is not comfortable or easy. You won't automatically have more energy nor will you always feel full every moment of the day. There is the reality of muscle soreness, occasional hunger, and just the drain of making a life change. But the sacrifices are well worth the effort. That's what you have to remind yourself about. I will say though that if you are working out regularly you will probably sleep very well at night. That's one immediately benefit.

Actually, it's all worth it because you will see results. Right now with a total loss of 31.9 pounds my clothes are too big. That's a good problem to have. I decide to visit a local alterations business to take in some of my clothes.

I'm only too happy to have my clothes taken in. That owner of the alteration's business is excited for me. She keeps saying "you're doing so well Monica". Well of course she's excited for me she's profiting as I'm losing weight. This means more business for her. But her encouragement means a lot.

In fact, encouragement is important along the RSYL journey. I'm thankful at this point that I have a few people in my life that encourage me and do not try to undermine my efforts. This will be an important factor to your success in the journey.

The bible teaches us that to find a faithful friend we must also be one. Be a faithful friend and pray for some faithful friends in your life. You will need them in the RSYL journey.

# WEIGHING IN AND WRITING IT DOWN

This journey requires persistence, courage and diligence. Make some notes below about how you're working to stay persistent, courageous and diligent. Also, record this month's weight loss and fitness goals, your progress, and challenges.

_____
_____
_____
_____
_____
_____
_____
_____
_____
_____
_____
_____
_____
_____
_____
_____
_____
_____
_____
_____
_____
_____
_____
_____
_____
_____
_____
_____

***Prayer*** Father, I ask you in Jesus Name to make me a person of persistence, courage, and diligence. Help me to see that I don't have to give up because of obstacles. Give me the grace to see myself as you see me. Give me the power to overcome and persist and achieve the goals I have set out to achieve. ***AMEN***

***Commit your actions to the Lord and your plans will succeed.***

***Proverbs 16:3 NLT***

# OVERVIEW OF MONTHS 6 & 7

The Big Picture

Confidence gained through discipline

***Weighing In Week # 22*** (-1.1 lbs)     ***Total Weight Loss 33. lbs.***

Now that I've lost over 30 pounds I definitely feel a sense of accomplishment. Literally, I feel differently. It's not just a matter of clothes being too big or others comments I feel differently. I understand on a more personal level the correlation between healthy eating choices and results on the scale. I have faced my fear of working out. I am starting to see the Big Picture. This is a pivotal moment for me and it will be for you too. The Big Picture brings the RSYL journey into proper perspective.

Most people live for the here and now. That's what our microwave generation does best. It's about right now – instant gratification and how does this whole thing make me feel? Successful people know it's good to recognize the here and now but we must also understand that there will be a later too.

That's what got Esau into trouble. Remember him the guy from the Bible? He lost his entire inheritance (birthright) I mean he gave it up willingly all for the here and now. He said in fact:

## Genesis 25:29-32 (NLT)

**One day when Jacob was cooking some stew, Esau arrived home**

**from the wilderness exhausted and hungry. 30 Esau said to Jacob, "I'm starved! Give me some of that red stew!" 31 "All right," Jacob replied, "but trade me your rights as the firstborn son." 32 "Look, I'm dying of starvation!" said Esau. "What good is my birthright to me now?"**

In other words, here's what happened. Esau came in tired and hungry (ever felt that way?). I mean he'd been outside working all day. He comes in to smell some very good stew. Ever notice how the scent of food fills a room and you just think "I am so hungry"?. That's how Esau felt.

Jacob said basically, yes I will give you some stew. Just give me your inheritance. This is a ludicrous proposition. Who would give up their entire lifetime of inheritance for a bowl of stew? But Esau did it. He was so tired and so hungry in the here and now he said – I am about to die just feed me. In other words, I don't care about tomorrow just give me food now !!!

This here and now attitude does not consider the big picture. As you RSYL take time to consider the big picture. It's not all about today. It's not all about giving up cookies, candy, fat laden and sugar soaked foods. It's about making healthy choices with right sized portions so that you will have a better tomorrow.

More and more as the Big Picture becomes clearer healthy choices today will become easier.

*Weighing In Week # 23* (-1.0 lbs)     *Total Weight Loss 34 lbs.*

I am so happy to see the number on the scale decrease. This doesn't get old for me.

*Weighing In Week # 24* (-1.0 lbs)     *Total Weight Loss 35 lbs.*

*Weighing In Week # 25* (- 1.6 lbs)     *Total Weight Loss 36.6 lbs.*

As I continue on this RSYL journey and the Big Picture continues to become clearer I realize that something really interesting has changed.

Prior to this journey I rarely ate breakfast. I didn't have the time I reasoned. I heard eating breakfast makes you hungrier all day (this is not true – this is a myth, fable etc). If I did eat breakfast it was a donut, pastry, or candy bar. Take your pick I like all three. I realized though that now I no longer walk around all day hungry or skipping meals.

Now, I want my sharing of this journey to be honest. I did experience moments of hunger on this year long RSYL journey. But the truth be told, prior to Right Sizing I was hungry a lot. I would on many occasions skip breakfast and lunch and by the time I'd get home I was so hungry for dinner. I was hungry enough for dinner that I didn't care what I ate – or how much. At this point I now realize that habit has changed completely. I realize that one of the keys to sticking with Right Sizing is that I never let myself get too hungry.

As a part of RSYL I eat breakfast. I also usually have a mid-morning snack (ex. fruit or vegetables). I eat a healthy right sized lunch. Sometimes, I have an afternoon snack of vegetables or fruit. This routine helps me to not overeat. I never have that feeling of "I am just so hungry I could eat anything".

That is essentially what happened to Esau. He let himself get so hungry he could no longer think straight. Yes, I know Esau had other problems. I have read about them in the bible. One of his issues though was that he didn't take care of himself on a continual basis. He would go out and work and not take time to nourish himself. Then he got so hungry one day that even his inheritance seemed to be of no value to him. The RSYL lesson here is: don't' let yourself get too hungry (unless you're fasting for spiritual reasons and that's a completely different matter entirely). Really hungry people don't usually make wise decisions. Really hungry people tend to make impetuous decisions.

As you RSYL make sure you keep yourself on a steady schedule. This is a part of seeing the Big Picture. If you don't let yourself get to the point of being too hungry you won't be as tempted to overeat. Strange as it sounds the very thing I feared would make me fat – eating 3 meals per day was the thing that actually helped me Right Size my life.

## THE BIG PICTURE IS KEY TO RSYL.

*Weighing In Week # 26* (- .6 **lbs**)　　　<u>*Total Weight Loss 37.2 lbs.*</u>

Slow week for weight loss. I'm not bothered by it this particular weigh in – apparently I am just having a really good day. I just stick with the food plan, the food journal and I keep on working out.

## WEIGHING IN AND WRITING IT DOWN

How are you working to keep in mind The Big Picture? Can you see in the past how maybe you did not consider the big picture - but only the "instant fix". Along with recording this months weight loss and fitness goals also take some time to journal about your big picture. Write down some specific ways you will guard against skipping meals and allowing yourself to get too hungry. If you get too hungry you'll be tempted to overeat. The big picture is key to RSYL.

---------------------------------------------------------------
---------------------------------------------------------------
---------------------------------------------------------------
---------------------------------------------------------------
---------------------------------------------------------------
---------------------------------------------------------------
---------------------------------------------------------------
---------------------------------------------------------------
---------------------------------------------------------------
---------------------------------------------------------------
---------------------------------------------------------------
---------------------------------------------------------------
---------------------------------------------------------------
---------------------------------------------------------------
---------------------------------------------------------------
---------------------------------------------------------------
---------------------------------------------------------------
---------------------------------------------------------------
---------------------------------------------------------------
---------------------------------------------------------------
---------------------------------------------------------------
---------------------------------------------------------------
---------------------------------------------------------------
---------------------------------------------------------------

*Prayer* - Father, teach me to guard against relying on the "quick fix" when it comes to losing weight or working out. Show me the benefits of the Big Picture and bring the Big Picture to my remembrance when I am tempted to think only of the "here and now". *AMEN*

### *Weighing In Week* # 27 (-2.0 lbs)    *Total Weight Loss 39.2 lbs.*

I'm excited I had a big loss this week. This is always good encouragement and incentive for me.

Previous to the RSYL journey I struggled with some areas of discipline in my life. Not in every area. I excelled in school. I was responsible at work. I was responsible at home.

Personally though, I lacked discipline. I did not make eating healthy food and working out a priority. As I'm on this journey I start to realize that I am developing discipline on a personal level. I mean I am starting to like the routine and structure. Don't misunderstand this is still a sacrifice. It doesn't always feel good. But I like the results and I like how it's changing me. Not just physically but personally and even spiritually.

I began to see the scripture "endure hardness as a good soldier" come to life for me. The truth is making right food choices and working out consistently is hard at times. What I found though is that as I continue on the path I am learning many things.

I am learning that I can do what's difficult if I persist. At first, I couldn't run for 30 minutes on the treadmill. I couldn't run at all. I couldn't keep up in any of the workout classes. I can now. That sense of accomplishment is not just some worldly "feel good" thing. This is what God intended for His people. This is a part of walking in dominion and power and under His authority. This is part of being effective and productive and understanding that you can achieve. In fact, as you continue on this journey you will eventually ask yourself why didn't I do this a long time ago? This is great !!!!

### *Weighing In Week # 28 (- 3.0 lbs)*      *Total Weight Loss 42.2 lbs.*

Losing 3 pounds in a week is huge for me. I celebrate this week as I am over the 40 pound loss mark !!

Lots of experts say that it's important to celebrate your successes. Certainly, I agree with that. I'm no expert in fitness or nutrition. But I am an expert in sticking with the RSYL process. Several times various groups have invited me to come and speak and share my weight loss journey in order to encourage people.

I'm always happy to do so.

Frequently, one of the questions is: "as I lose weight should I reward myself with food"? Really, you have to make your own decision about that. Personally, I did not do that. The reward for me was the weight loss, the smaller size clothing, the sense of growing stronger, or even a manicure, or a massage. But not food. I'm really not sure how eating a slice of chocolate cake is a reward for losing just over 40 pounds.

I would suggest finding other non-food related ways to celebrate your weight loss success. Specifically, ways that don't have the potential the pack the pounds back on.

### *Weighing In Week # 29 (-1.2 lbs)*      *Total Weight Loss 43.4 lbs.*

### *Weighing In Week # 30 (- 2.0 lbs)*      *Total Weight Loss 45.4 lbs.*

### *Weighing In Week # 31 (- 1.8 lbs)*      *Total Weight Loss 47.2lbs.*

As I approach the almost 50 pounds of weight loss mark I am so excited that I just can't stand it. I've had to give away more clothes, have more clothes altered and buy new stuff than I would have ever imagined. I wouldn't trade it for anything though. It's been a hard but exciting journey.

Obviously for everyone on the RSYL journey there are different and varying amounts of weight to be lost. At some point though, in the weight loss journey you will start to receive compliments on your progress. But you may say that sounds wonderful. It is wonderful. Yes it is. It may also cause you to feel somewhat uncomfortable – or not.

There came a point for me that it got uncomfortable. It was uncomfortable for many different reasons. Sometimes I felt pressured. I would think – can I keep this up? What if I mess up and gain it all back? That would be embarrassing. I had never stuck with any diet this long. Would I mess up?

I mention this because it's part of the journey. In all likelihood there may be a moment that you just think "I am afraid I will put the weight back on". I am NOT speaking this on you – this is NOT a negative confession. This may happen in your human experience. This type of thought, fear worry, concern is NOT from God and you don't have to tolerate it.

If this happens, go back to the section on Clearing the Clutter. Clear the clutter out of your thought life. Admit in prayer to God what you're feeling and what you fear. Everyone and I mean everyone that is living and breathing has been afraid of one thing or another in life. God hasn't given us a spirit of fear but let's face it sometimes fear presents itself. You don't have to hang out there.

You can shed fear by renewing your mind in God's truth. As people give you compliments thank God for your progress. He's helped you this far and He will continue to do so.

*"If you fail under pressure, your strength is too small."*

*Proverbs 24:10 NLT*

# WEIGHING IN AND WRITING IT DOWN

How are you doing in terms of renewing your mind in the truth? Have you been clearing the clutter on a daily basis? If not, write down a specific plan to clear the clutter. Perhaps you can set aside 5 minutes each day to read scripture and clear your mind of negative thoughts. Also, write down your weight loss, fitness goals and progress.

***Prayer*** - Father, help me to renew my mind in your Word. I want to clear the clutter from my mind and meditate on what you say about me and about my life. I pray all negativity is gone and replaced with the goodness of your Word. Bring your Word to my remembrance whenever I am tempted to think on negative thoughts. ***AMEN***

# OVERVIEW OF MONTHS 8 & 9

Dealing with myriad of personal questions

Help, I've become the center of attention!

*__Weighing In Week # 32__* (-1.0 lbs)     <u>*__Total Weight Loss 48.2lbs.__*</u>

One day I'm out with my husband. We were out having a perfectly good time. Out of nowhere a man and a lady walk up to us. The man says "Monica, you look so beautiful. You've lost so much weight. How much do you weigh now?"

In all likelihood this man had seen me on television. I'm sure that probably exacerbated the situation. He felt like "he knew me well enough to ask". I don't feel like anyone knows anyone well enough to ask this particular question – but apparently this man felt differently.

This was the first of many uncomfortable situations for me. Chances are you will encounter on your RSYL journey some out of line questions. I want you to be prepared in advance. If you want to answer then go ahead. If you're like me you don't want to answer.

So what's a girl or guy to do? Laugh. Make a joke. I said things like if I answered that question for you I'd have to ship you off to Siberia or some remote place later to make sure my secret is safe. (I was kidding of course). The idea here is to guard your heart and make yourself comfortable. Some people just have "foot in mouth" disease and they just don't know when to "be quiet".

*Weighing In Week # 33* (-1.0 lbs)   <u>*Total Weight Loss 49.2lbs.*</u>

*Weighing In Week # 34* (- 2.0 lbs)   <u>*Total Weight Loss 51.2lbs.*</u>

Okay so 50 pounds are off now and it feels wonderful. About now I do have more energy. Yes, I am still sore and tired on occasion but overall physically I feel like a different person.

The closer you get to your goal weight the more compliments and comments you will receive from other people. Some of these comments may cause you to fear and think what if I gain it all back? Others comments may make you feel uncomfortable and wish you weren't getting so much attention.

Getting all that attention can be an uncomfortable situation. While we understand that our entire life is not about our outer appearance (and it's not). We live in a world consumed with outer appearance. Youth, beauty, and thinness are celebrated in this culture. Let's face it sometimes these attributes are "overly" celebrated in the church too.

With that in mind let's approach this subject honestly. There were various points in my RSYL journey that I just thought seriously? Seriously, all this hoopla over weight loss? I mean let's just be honest about this in my life I have faced many things. I have faced serious things like betrayal and come to a place of forgiveness of hope and never received such admiration from onlookers. For whatever reason it seems that weight loss is just highly celebrated. It may also be uncomfortable because when you're struggling with excess weight you're usually working to hide it. Now in the weight loss process your progress is highly visible. People see the losses and they can't help but talk about it.

*"Be who you are and say what you feel, because those who mind don't matter and those who matter don't mind."*

**~Dr. Seuss**

If it feels uncomfortable to be the seeming "center of attention" this is something to pray about and work through. It can be done. I did it and sometimes still have to do it. That's right these things have a way of "coming back". Handle the compliments and comments as graciously as you can and prayerfully handle giving any of it too much credit in your life.

### I Samuel 16:7 NLT

**The LORD doesn't see things the way you see them. People judge by outward appearance, but the LORD looks at the heart.".**

# WEIGHING IN AND WRITING IT DOWN

Record below how you're making an effort to renew your mind and clear the clutter. By this time, you may have already started receiving compliments on your weight loss. How are you handling that? Is it throwing you off track. In your RSYL plan make sure you renewing your mind and praying about this journey on a regular basis. Also, record this months weight loss and fitness goals, your progress, and challenges. If you list a challenge make sure you write down some specific ways to overcome.

_____

_____

_____

_____

_____

_____

_____

_____

_____

_____

_____

_____

_____

_____

_____

_____

_____

_____

_____

_____

_____

_____

_____

***Prayer*** - Father I ask that you help me be so rooted and grounded in you that I do not give anyone words (compliments or not) too much place in my life. Father, help me to have my identity solely in you. Let me experience true freedom through your Word. ***AMEN***

*Weighing In Week # 35 (- 2.2 lbs)*    *Total weight Loss 53.4 lbs.*

As you RSYL you're expending a lot of energy to become healthier. That's important and of great value. At the same time our character and the issues of our heart are most important. As you are on the RSYL journey and making so many adjustments and learning new healthy habits also pray continually for the character of Christ to be formed in you. That is after all the ultimate goal for every follower of Christ.

*Weighing In Week # 36 (-1.8 lbs)*    *Total Weight Loss 55.2lbs.*

*Weighing In Week # 37 (- .2 lbs)*    *Total Weight Loss 55.4 lbs.*

I am a little tired of this right now. I know I have had some good losses for the last few weeks but losing .2 pounds in one week? I know. I know. Why whine when you've lost just over 50 pounds? It's like this sometimes when you RSYL.

Sometimes it's aggravating. Other times it's exciting. Sometimes you are just like – I want this to be over. Be prepared for these moments while you are on your journey. It's all a part of the process.

*Weighing In Week # 38 (- 1.0 lbs)*    *Total Weight Loss 56.4 lbs.*

*Weighing In Week # 39 (-1.0 lbs.*    *Total Weight Loss 57.4 lbs.*

# WEIGHING IN

Is it ever uncomfortable for you to be receiving attention over your weight loss? This journal is an opportunity to be honest and address these situations. They won't just go away. It's also an opportunity to keep in mind that everything is not about outer appearance. Our inner character is also of the utmost importance. Challenge yourself to keep the right priorities and balance as you move forward in RSYL. Record this months weight loss and fitness goals, your progress, and challenges.

_____

_____

_____

_____

_____

_____

_____

_____

_____

_____

_____

_____

_____

_____

_____

_____

_____

_____

_____

_____

_____

_____

**Prayer** - Father I pray to be conformed into the image of your Son Jesus Christ. I ask that my inner character would be a reflection of your son. Make me rich in mercy and gentle with all so that the love of Christ will be evident in my life. Thank you for helping me to Right Size My Life. Help me to stay on this journey and bless and prosper the work of my hands. *AMEN*

# OVERVIEW OF MONTHS 10 & 11

Are we there yet?

My sister asks me to run a ½ marathon with her

Helping Overweight Children

The holidays are coming

***Weighing In Week # 40 (- .2 lbs)***     ***Total Weight Loss 57.6lbs.***

After stepping on the scale this week I wanted to say "are we there yet?" Obviously, I am not there yet. I wish I was that's for sure. When I started this RSYL journey I thought for sure I would be at goal weight right now. I'm glad I didn't know when I get started how long it would take.

I started in January and finishing in September sounded like a good long time. Now I realize it will be December or perhaps a little longer. I feel like that little child a long car ride saying, "are we there yet"?

> *"Quit now, you'll never make it. If you disregard this advice, you'll be halfway there."*
>
> ~David Zucker

***Weighing In Week # 41***   **(-1.0 lbs)**     ***Total weight Loss 58.6lbs.***

***Weighing In Week # 42*** **(-.4 lbs)**     ***Total Weight Loss 59 lbs.***

I talk to my sister today and tell her about my progress. My sister has always been thin. She's consistently made healthy food choices. She's an avid runner too. Did I mention that? I've always been close to my sister and I've always admired her healthy lifestyle.

I am glad to share my good news about my weight loss with her. She's excited for me. I also tell her how I've been working out on a regular basis. At this point she invites me to train to run a ½ marathon with her. I balk of course, Who in the world – I mean what normal, average person runs a ½ marathon? Now I realize that all kinds of normal everyday people run ½ marathons. At the time though I thought that only the finest of athletes attempted such great feats.

She says I can do it. She sends me the training schedule. I say okay. I'll try. This something I would have never committed to in the past. One thing that regular work outs will teach you is that God designed your body to move. We were never intended to be sedentary creatures. In other words, being a couch potato is not really in the "abundant life plan".

I set out to see if I can keep the ½ marathon training schedule.

# WEIGHING IN AND WRITING IT DOWN

Does it seem like this journey is the trip that will never end? Write about it. Remind yourself of your goals and what this process is teaching you. As you record this months weight loss and fitness goals go back over your previous journal entries and see how far you've come. In all likelihood, you've made a lot of progress and don't want to get off track now.

_____

_____

_____

_____

_____

_____

_____

_____

_____

_____

_____

_____

_____

_____

_____

_____

_____

_____

_____

_____

_____

_____

_____

_____

***Prayer*** - Father give me everything I need to stay the course. I pray for patience during this journey and encouragement along this road. I thank you for being close to me through this process. Let me sense your presence in a greater way. Open my eyes to see the benefits in this journey and the benefits of serving you and staying faithful. ***AMEN***

*Weighing In Week # 43* (- 1.0 lbs)    *Total Weight Loss 60lbs.*

*Weighing In Week # 44* (-1.2 lbs)    *Total of Weight Loss 61.2lbs.*

Are we there yet? Will we ever get there?

*Weighing In Week # 45* (-1.2 lbs)    **Total Weight Loss 62.4.lbs.**

As I start out on the ½ marathon training schedule I think a lot about my sister. I think about her healthy and active lifestyle. I always admired that about her. As I review my RSYL journey and family of origin. I realize once again that I was the only person in my family that was overweight as a child.

I remember how difficult that was for me in some ways. Now the percentage of overweight children is climbing at an alarming rate. Back in the day though overweight children were few and far between. I can clearly remember thinking that I was the only "chubby kid" in school.

I was certainly the only chubby kid in my family. My family tried very hard to help me with my weight problem. Even the doctor suggested many diets. I just couldn't/wouldn't stick with them. There was always junk food in the house and I loved junk food. I did feel very badly about my weight problem. I felt badly enough to cry about. I felt badly enough to sit out certain activities. I could not however overcome the weight problem.

If you're reading this right now and you have a child or children that are overweight the best thing that you can do is be a good example. Further, fill your house with nourishing, healthy food choices. The next helpful thing that you can do is get outside with your child and be as active as you can. Focusing on your child's weight problem – teasing your child about their weight problem will not work. You also need to protect your child from other well-meaning family members; friends etc. that say mean and negative things to your child. These comments are not helpful. They in fact damage your child. Don't allow it.

I understand that some children (adults too) can eat unhealthy junk food and stay thin. That's not the point or the issue here. The point is not everyone can do that. The next point is even if they can do that and remain thin – it's still not healthy. Healthy living is the point. Fill your home with healthy nourishing food and an active lifestyle. This will reduce and eliminate the overweight issue in many cases.

If you are the parent you have control of the home environment and you can set the stage for your child's success.

*Weighing In Week # 46* (-1.0 lbs)       *Total Weight Loss 63.4lbs.*

At this point I am so glad I decided to Right Size my Life. I run across a quote by Henry David Thoreau it says:

**"Men were born to succeed, not to fail".**

I think that's some good inspiration. That's what God promises that He has good plans for us.

**Jeremiah 29:11.**

**For I know the plans I have for you," says the LORD. "They are plans for good and not for disaster, to give you a future and a hope.**

*Weighing In Week # 47* (-1.0 lbs)       *Total Weight Loss  64.4lbs.*

*Weighing In Week # 48* (- 2.0 lbs)       *Total Weight Loss  66.4lbs.*

At this point, I am working on purchasing a whole new wardrobe. This is a wonderful problem to have. I used to hate shopping. I couldn't ever find anything to fit properly. Now everything fits. Now I have to guard against the desire to buy everything in the store.

No one can believe that I love shopping. I think of reasons to go shopping. I have had my old clothes altered and re-altered enough. It's time for new. It's time for shopping.

I learn something astounding at this juncture in the RSYL journey. My entire life people said to me you are not fat just "big boned". You have a large frame. Why do people feel like they need to make comments? There is not a real answer to that question. I pose it just because I wonder. That used to make me feel so badly. I felt especially badly because my mom and sister are thin and petite. I discovered in my shopping journey that I wore a size 4 Petite. Honestly, I couldn't believe it.

In fact, I drove to 3 different stores that day just to confirm my findings. When I went into each store I fully expected to find out that I was wrong. I did not think I could wear a size 4 Petite for real. But I did. When I looked in the mirror I could tell that I had lost weight. I never thought though that I could wear that particular size.

I believed what I had been told my whole life. I had been told that I was big and that I had a large frame and yet this wasn't true. We've all been told things by people (even people that love us) that just aren't true. It can take awhile for us to get to the place where that lie is exposed.

This is a part of the renewing of your mind process. This is a process that is a part of the believer's daily life. Every day we have to clear the clutter.

Even when you get to your goal weight (and as you keep at it you will). You will still need to renew your mind. You will still need to guard your heart against the lies of the world, your flesh and the enemy. The good news is though that you can do it.

*"You can always do more than you think you can"*.

**Bobbi Mofield, Personal Trainer Extraordinaire, Sports Village**

# WEIGHING IN AND WRITING IT DOWN

Perhaps you've set a fitness goal that is or seemed like the "impossible dream". Record that goal below and list specific ways that you plan to achieve it. Break it down into smaller segments that will help it be more achievable. Continue to use the journal below to record your weight loss efforts and achievements. If there is an area in which you are struggling write it down and think about how you can put that difficulty behind you.

_____

_____

_____

_____

_____

_____

_____

_____

_____

_____

_____

_____

_____

_____

_____

_____

_____

_____

_____

_____

_____

_____

_____

**Prayer** - Father I thank you that you promised that all things are possible for those who believe. I believe in you and I ask you to lead me in the process and show me how to reach my goals. Give me a willing heart and spirit to do my part on this journey. Show me how to be diligent in all matters. Let me experience success your way. ***AMEN***

# THE FINAL FOUR

*Weighing In Week # 49* (- 2.0 lbs)    *Total Weight Loss  68.4lbs.*

This entire RSYL journey is about how you can do it.  It may be slow (or not) but whatever the case this is a journey that you can complete. This is a track in life that you can run and keep at it.  As you come to the end of the weight loss portion of the journey keep in mind all of the effort that it took to get there.  Cherish the progress and the lessons that you've learned.

Write down the lessons that were most helpful to you.  There's a power in writing things down.   There's something about the written word that's permanent and powerful.   Review what you've written time and time again.  Sometimes I just go back through my written journal just to remember and also to celebrate.  It's easy to forget "where you came from".  Don't let that happen.  Remind yourself of the progress and the hard work.  This will help you to never go back to unhealthy habits. After all, the RSYL journey is a lifestyle and you've come to far now to go back.

# WEIGHING IN AND WRITING IT DOWN

At this point in your RSYL journey you have learned some major lessons. It's important to understand all that you've learned as it will help you appreciate the process. Record some of the most important lessons you learned. Think about how those lessons will help you in your personal and/or professional life.

_____

_____

_____

_____

_____

_____

_____

_____

_____

_____

_____

_____

_____

_____

_____

_____

_____

_____

_____

_____

_____

_____

_____

_____

_____

_____

*Prayer* - Father help me to have a teachable spirit. Thank you for all I am learning on this journey. Keep my heart pliable and open to your ways. Teach me all that you desire for me to know. My heart and life are open to you. *AMEN*

*Weighing In Week # 50 (- .2 lbs)*      *Total Weight Loss  68.6lbs.*

At this point I love shopping and I also love working out. Weighing in is not such an issue for me anymore. My trainer is totally excited for me. He starts giving me the "holiday advice". I needed the holiday advice too. I just kept thinking there is no way I will gain an ounce during the holidays.

In fact, I stepped up my workouts during the month of November and December. I did though allow myself to eat a great Thanksgiving Dinner and Christmas dinner. When I say great though I do not mean that I allowed myself to overeat. I did not. Don't you do that either. You will be sorry if you do that.

You can't let your progress go to waste. Bring all of your RSYL choices to the table for the Holidays. Go back to the section on portions. Divide up that plate. Allow yourself something that's special for the holiday. But you don't have to overdo it. In fact, you'll be a whole lot happier if you don't overdo it. Make sure to stay physically active during the holidays too. Working out is a great tool to the management of your weight.

> *"If you're enjoying this fitness class tell a friend- if you're not enjoying it please don't tell anyone."*

**Bobbi Mofield, Personal Trainer Extraordinaire, Sport Village**

*Weighing In Week # 51  (- .2 lbs)*      *Total Weight Loss 68.8lbs.*

I know almost only counts in horseshoes….but I am almost there !!!

*Weighing In Week # 52 (-1.0 lbs)*      *Total Weight Loss  69.8lbs.*

Goal weight finally !!!!! I believed it and I couldn't believe it. Other than the day I got married and the day I had my son I have never been happier. This was the hardest work I had ever done. This was harder for me than graduating from college or any other task I could recall.

I celebrated with a veggie burger, pita pocket, lots of mustard, onions, and an apple. This was my favorite RSYL dinner at that time. For dessert I enjoyed a Weight Watcher key lime pie dessert. I record all of it in my food journal which I keep to this day.

# WEIGHING IN AND WRITING IT DOWN

Perhaps you've met your weight loss and fitness goals - if so, congratulations. Use the space below to record your biggest challenges and successes. This will be important to you later when you are in the maintenance phase. It's always good to see how far you've come and it will help you to never look back.

_____

_____

_____

_____

_____

_____

_____

_____

_____

_____

_____

_____

_____

_____

_____

_____

_____

_____

_____

_____

_____

_____

_____

_____

_____

_____

_____

_____

_____

**Prayer** - Father thank you for allowing me to come this far. Thank you for courage and strength to run this race. Father give me the ability to continue on this path. Let me see everything I've learned through this journey through your eyes. Thank you Father for granting me success. Everything good and perfect thing that I have Father has come from you. *AMEN*

# MAINTENANCE

This is the moment you've been waiting for. Celebrate to its' fullest. You have the lost the weight you set out to lose and you will not regain it if you follow the maintenance phase of your weight reduction plan. For me this phase was the easiest. That's right I said the easiest. After all I had been developing healthy eating habits and consistently working out for one entire year. Now was the time to transition from weight loss mode to maintenance mode. The maintenance phase is critical to your long term success.

The Weight Watcher maintenance phase lasts for 6 weeks. The good news is you'll get to eat just a little bit more now. Isn't that good news? Your maintenance plan will guide you through adding some extra food items over time. If for some reason your weight reduction plan does not have a maintenance plan consult with a health care professional or nutritionist immediately. They are knowledgeable and can help you through this final phase. You have invested a lot of time energy and effort and this is not the time to stop. You are setting the stage right now for your long term success.

You'll still need a food journal. I still keep a food journal now. I write down everything I eat. It's for my own records. It helps me keep track. I'm so happy to have lost all that weight that recording what I eat each day is a small, small task. I don't mind at all. Follow the prescribed maintenance eating plan carefully. It is your key to success. Stick with the good habits you've developed over the journey.

While on the maintenance phase you'll want to continue working out (if you've been working out). I found the 6 weeks to be a delight. I was amazed at how the weight was staying off. The thing is the more slowly you lose the weight the easier it is to keep it off.

# WEIGHING IN - THE MAINTENANCE PHASE

The maintenance phase - was it easier or harder than you expected? Can you believe you've come this far? Record your fears and dreams about being in this phase. Write down how important it is to you to continue along this path and not get distracted. Write down specifically what you will do if you find yourself getting off track. Remember you've come to far now to go back !!! Congratulations.

_____
_____
_____
_____
_____
_____
_____
_____
_____
_____
_____
_____
_____
_____
_____
_____
_____
_____
_____
_____
_____
_____
_____
_____
_____

**Prayer** - Father thank you for allowing me to Right Size my life. I pray you will continue to give me strength and grace to walk out on a daily basis all I have learned on this journey. I thank you Father that you have brought me this far and that you will continue to be with me and give me all that I need. Thank you Father - you are good and I know your plans for me are good. Let me walk in your good plan for me today and every day. **AMEN**

# RSYL LIFESTYLE

Your new RSYL eating and working out have paid off. This is now your new healthy lifestyle. I still go to the monthly Weight Watcher meetings. I am a lifetime member. The sense of belonging and community help me. Most plans offer some type of follow-up. Keep with that follow-up as it will help you.

I have kept the weight off for over 3 years. It has not been a problem for me. While I was on the journey my lifestyle changed. That's the key. I used to think how awful when people said you will have to watch what you eat for your whole life. I used to just think I want this weight problem to go away. The truth is with healthy eating habits and an active lifestyle the weight does go away over time. What we're left with at the end of the journey is a new lifestyle. A lifestyle that nourishes us and creates the best scenario for our nutritional and physical health.

You aren't giving up anything when you RSYL. You are receiving such benefit. By now on this journey you will have more energy. You will feel better and look better. You will have more confidence. As you've prayed through this journey you have learned how God delights in the details of your life.

You've gained discipline and courage. After all you've faced something significant and conquered. Yes, it's God that gives us victory. But we have to make decisions and do the right things along the way too.

There are definitely some key ingredients to Right Sizing Your Life. Those key ingredients include right sizing your portions, working out consistently, keeping a food journal and praying through your journey. These are all a part of the lifestyle and should not be neglected now that you've reached weight.

One biblical principle that comes to mind is "counting the cost". That's essential in making any changes to your lifestyle. Think about all the hard work you've done so far. You've made and kept a commitment to lose weight, change your eating habits and work out. All of these things cost – whether it's time or money or both they cost. Now that you are at goal weight keep the cost in mind. The more you keep the cost mind the less likely you are to turn back on the journey.

Think about it if you purchase a very expensive home, car, or piece of property chances are you are not going to just "abandon it". You are going to do what it takes to maintain the investment. It's the same thing on the Right Sizing Your Life Journey. You've invested time, money, and effort and you don't want to let that go. You want to continue practicing the same good habits that got you to goal weight.

A healthy lifestyle is lived just one day at a time. Just one good decision at a time. You can continue living your new healthy lifestyle and enjoying the benefits. You have accomplished so much and have so much to be thankful about. You are someone that has proven themselves diligent and consistent. These are traits required for success.

> *"If we did the things we are capable of, we would astound ourselves."*
> **~Thomas Edison**

Congratulations. I am proud of you. Write and tell me about your story at www.monicaspeaks.com

# BASIC NUTRITION

I can remember growing up that most people talked about the four basic food groups. They included protein (mostly meats), breads/grains, /fruits, /vegetables, and dairy products. As the science of nutrition has grown so have the food groups. There is much more information available today about healthy eating and dietary plans.

That's why it's important for you to consult with an expert about your food plan. Your specific calorie intake and servings per day will vary according to many different factors. Some of those factors include age, height, weight, gender, and physical activity level. You will need to learn especially as you are Right Sizing what your proper caloric intake is to lose weight and then what it will be when you're on the maintenance plan. Other than your personal nutritional plan you food journal will be your next best friend. Learn all you can about nutrition as knowledge is power. Your choices will be better choices simply because you are informed about your good health.

I learned many things about nutrition and losing weight as I traveled on the RSYL journey. I read nutrition labels now and make my eating decisions based on what those labels say. I will share in this next section some basic shopping tips for the best nutrition. I will also share some of my favorite healthy recipe and dinner ideas.

# RSYL FOOD SHOPPING TIPS FOR BASIC MEATS

Protein is an important part of any healthy eating plan. Your specific eating plan will outline the proper number of portions each day. Protein is especially important for you if you are doing any kind of weight training in your work out.

**Lean Beef** - *the leanest cuts of beef include tenderloin and top sirloin. To keep beef moist, try sautéing it quickly over high heat.*

*Nutrition facts for 3-ounce serving: 165 Calories, 25 g protein, 0 G carbohydrate, 7 g fat, 2.5g saturated fat, 0 g fiber.*

**Fish -** *shop for fish that is firm and whose skin is translucent. If it smells, well, fishy, it's already starting to go bad. Fresh fish should be used or frozen within two days. Once in the freezer, it will keep for about a month.*

*Nutrition facts per 3- ounce serving: 119 Calories, 23 g protein, 0 g carbohydrate, 2.5 g fat 0 g saturated fat, 0 g fiber.*

**Chicken** - *Place chicken breasts between two sheets of plastic wrap and gently pound with a tenderizer until they are of uniform thickness. This will ensure even cooking.*

*Nutrition facts per 3-ounce serving: 142 calories, 27 g protein, 0 g carbohydrate, 3 g fat 1 g saturated fat, 0 g fiber.*

**Lean Ground Turkey** - *To cut calories and fat, look for packages containing all white meat. Feeding a big crew? Stretch your turkey- and money-by mixing it with 10% Grape-Nuts cereal.*

*Nutrition facts per 3-ounce serving: 145 calories, 17 g protein, 0 g carbohydrates, 8 g fat, 2 g saturated, 0 g fiber.*

Most experts in nutrition say that you should eat 1 serving of a complete protein within one hour of working out particularly if you are doing weight training. Eating protein helps rebuild your muscles.

### *RSYL Fruit and Veggie Info*

### *"Eat your fruits and vegetables – they are good for you."*

### *Mom.*

Once I learned to enjoy fruits and vegetables and incorporate them into my everyday eating plan I was able to stay full much more easily. I pray it will be the same for you. As I expanded my food repertoire to include fresh fruits and veggies I made it a point to learn about their nutritional value and caloric count. Some of the things I learned really surprised me.

About Potatoes

For example, I would frequently hear people say when you wanted to lose weight you could not eat potatoes and lose weight. I had always heard it said that potatoes are fattening. The truth is a loaded baked potato (butter, cheese bacon and sour cream) is not a wise weight loss choice. But a plain potato (medium sized) has only 110 calories, is naturally fat free, high in vitamin C and packs more potassium than a banana. I know you may be thinking but who eats a plain baked potato? I do and they're very delicious. It will be an adjustment at first but I promise as you continue on this path you taste buds will change and you'll find out that a plain potato (you can season to taste) is quite delicious and can be a very healthful choice for your weight loss plan.

About Spinach

Other than spinach being a "Popeye" favorite I was totally unfamiliar with spinach. Spinach is loaded with B vitamins and antioxidants that fight heart disease. They are also high in iron and dietary fiber and all kinds of things that are good for you. Additionally, they are very low in calories a mere 7 for one cup. No wonder Popeye loved spinach so much. See the recipe for the Strawberry Spinach salad and enjoy !

## About Onions

I was certainly aware that right after eating onions brushing and flossing was a must - what I didn't know was that onions are actually good for you. They are high in vitamin C and potassium. One cup of chopped onions have about 64 calories and 2.7 g of fiber. So onions are good for us but we still need to brush and floss right after eating.

## About Broccoli

I was familiar with hollandaise sauce and how fattening that was.... but broccoli? One cup of chopped broccoli has only 30 calories and is a good source of dietary fiber Broccoli is also very filling so start out eating your vegetables and you'll get full on fewer calories.

## About Green Beans

One 4 oz serving of green beans has only 40 calories and is a good source of dietary fiber. They are also a good source of vitamins A and C. When it comes to green beans you can enjoy and be guilt free !

## About Carrots

I had heard that carrots improve your eye sight what I hadn't heard was that they are high in vitamins A, B6, and C and have only 52 calories in one cup. Fresh carrots make a really good mid morning or afternoon snack.

## About Tomatoes

High in vitamins A and C and a good source of dietary fiber. Calorie count for 1 serving is low at a whopping 27 calories. They also taste good and are excellent on sandwiches and salads.

About Apples

I definitely knew that an apple a day would "keep the doctor away". Frequently, I would joke and say that two apples a day keeps the "specialist away". Seriously though apples are delicious and a mere 65 calories with 3 g of fiber (medium sized apple)

About Bananas

I heard many people talk about how bananas have a lot of calories. A small banana has 72 calories and is an excellent source of potassium. Bananas are one of my favorite fruits. Bananas are also an excellent snack and good in oatmeal.

About Grapes

1 cup of grapes totals 62 calories. Grapes are also low in saturated fat and high manganese. Plus they taste great and help fill you up. Try the turkey grape salad recipe. It is excellent for lunch or dinner.

About Oranges

Oranges are very high in vitamin C and 1 cup equals 85 calories. They are also high in potassium and high in thiamin.

About Pineapples

Pineapples have no cholesterol and are high in dietary fiber. Besides serving as a beautiful Hawaiian reminder they are high in thiamin and they are also excellent off the grill with chicken or steak.

About Blueberries

This low calorie natural snack contains antioxidants that help fight inflammation and lower bad LDL cholesterol, blood fats and blood sugar.

This is obviously not a comprehensive list of fruits and vegetables but the point is clear. Fresh fruits and veggies are an essential part of the Right Sizing Your life journey. If you don't like them - learn to like them. If you only like them drenched in butter and fancy cheese sauces - take the RSYL challenge to enjoy them plain. It will take a few weeks but you'll find that the effort is worth it. The fresh fruits and veggies will help fill you up and will add necessary vitamins to your daily eating regime.

In any grocery store most of the health filled foods are on the outer perimeter of the grocery store. Avoid the center aisles. They are usually loaded with empty calories, lots of sugar and lots of fat. The more you RSYL the less shopping you will do in the center aisles. Remember it's best to steer clear of temptation. If you just don't go down the cookie aisle you won't end up with cookies in your cupboard. Stick with the produce, meats/beans for protein, multi-grain breads, calcium rich foods like yogurt and milk.

In the next section of RSYL you'll find some dinner recipe ideas that are all high in protein, low in calories and low in fat. They are also easy to prepare and most can be made ahead in order to accommodate your busy schedule. Most importantly the dinner recipe ideas are all very good and tasty (I've tried them all).

It's important on the RSYL journey to make meal time healthy, delicious, fun and varied. These recipe ideas will help you do just that. You'll eat well and lose weight. It doesn't get better than that when you are on a RSYL journey.

# RSYL DINNER RECIPE IDEAS

All of these recipes are tried and true. They are healthy, delicious and low in fat. They can fit right into your RSYL journey.

## LAMB CHOPS WITH TOMATO CHUTNEY

Prep Time 15 Min     Cook 15 Min   Serves 4

| | |
|---|---|
| 4 | tsp olive oil |
| ½ | c. chopped onion |
| 2 | garlic cloves, minced |
| 4 | small plum tomatoes, chopped |
| ½ | cup diced orange bell pepper |
| ½ | tsp. sugar |
| ¼ | tsp. salt |
| ¼ | tsp. black pepper |
| 2 | Tbsp. minced fresh mint |
| 2 | Tbsp. lime juice |
| 1/8 | tsp. red pepper sauce |
| 4 | (4oz) trimmed loin lamb chops ¾ inch thick. |

Preheat the grill to medium or prepare a medium fire.

Meanwhile to make the chutney, heat the oil in a medium nonstick

Skillet over medium-high heat.  Add the onion and garlic; cook, stirring

Frequently, until softened, about 2 minutes.  Add the tomatoes, bell pepper,

Sugar, salt, and pepper; cook, stirring, until the bell pepper is crisp-tender, about 3 minutes.  Transfer the vegetable mixture to a small bowl.  Stir in the mint, lime juice, and pepper sauce; set aside.

Place the lamb chops on the grill rack and grill until an instant thermometer inserted into the thickest part of each chop registers 145 degrees for medium, about 5 minutes on each side. Transfer the lamb to a platter and serve topped with the chutney.

Per Serving (1 Lamb Chop with ½ c. chutney) 245 calories, 13 G FAT, 4 G SAT FAT, 0 G Trans FAT, 81 MG CHOL, 211 MG SOD, 5 G CARB, 1 G FIB, 26 G PROT, 29 MG CALC.

## CHICKEN ROLLS WITH TOMATO COMPOTE

Prep Time 20 Min      Cook 20 Min           Serves 4

| | |
|---|---|
| 1 | (6oz) bag baby spinach |
| 1 | tsp. olive oil |
| ½ | red onion, chopped |
| 1 | pint grape or cherry tomatoes halved |
| ¼ | tsp salt |
| 1 | tsp. balsamic vinegar |
| 2oz. | Reduced-fat black pepper goat cheese crumbled |
| ¼ | c. sun dried tomatoes (not packed in oil) chopped |
| 4 | (3oz) chicken cutlets |
| ½ | c. reduced sodium chicken broth |

Bring 1 inch of water to a boil in a large saucepan.  Add half the spinach and cook, stirring constantly, just until wilted, about 30 seconds.  Transfer with a slotted spoon to a colander.  Repeat with the remaining spinach.  Let cool and then squeeze dry.

To make the tomato compote head the oil in a large saucepan over medium heat. Add the red onion and cook, stirring occasionally, until softened, 5 minutes. Stir in the grape tomatoes and salt; cook, stirring occasionally, until the tomatoes begin to soften, about 2 minutes. Stir in the vinegar and set aside.

Mix the cheese and sun-dried tomatoes in a small bowl. Place the cutlets on a sheet of plastic wrap with the wind ends facing you. Working with a 1 cutlet at a time, place one fourth of the spinach in a line down the center of the cutlet leaving a ¾ inch border along the long sides; place one fourth of the cheese mixture at the wide end, roll up and secure with a toothpick. Repeat with the remaining cutlets, spinach, and cheese mixture to make 4 rolls.

Spray a medium nonstick skillet with nonstick spray and set over medium heat. Add the rolls and cook, turning occasionally, until browned, 5-6 minutes. Add the broth and bring to a boil. Reduce the heat and cook, covered, turning occasionally, until the rolls are cooked through about 7 minutes. Transfer the rolls with a slotted spoon to a cutting board; cover loose with foil and keep warm.

Bring the pan juices to a boil and cook until reduced to 3 Tbsp., about 1 minutes. Stir in the reserved tomato compote; reduce the head and cook until heated through.

To serve, remove the toothpicks from the rolls and cut each roll into 3 slices. Serve topped with the tomato compote.

Per Serving (3 slices with scant ½ c. compote) 196 Calories, 7 G Fat, 3 G SAT FAT, 0 G TRANS FAT, 58 MG CHOL, 425 MG SOD, 9 G CARB, 3 G FIB, 24 G PROT, 90 MG CALC.

# DOUBLE-TOMATO RISOTTO WITH SALMON

Prep Time 20 Min      Cook 25 Min      Serves 4

| | |
|---|---|
| 1 | (¾-lb) skinless salmon fillet |
| 1 | tsp. salt |
| 2-½ | c. reduced-sodium chicken broth |
| 1 | tsp. olive oil |
| 1 | onion, chopped |
| 1 | c. Arborio rice |
| 1 | large garlic clove, minced |
| 1 | zucchini, diced |
| 1 | c. shredded carrot |
| 1 | (¾-lb) beefsteak tomato, diced |
| ½ | c. tomato-vegetable juice |
| ¼ | tsp. black pepper |
| 3 | Tbsp. snipped fresh chives |

Place the salmon on a microwavable plate and sprinkle with ¼ tsp. of the salt. Cover with plastic wrap; then prick a few holes in the plastic. Microwave on Medium just until opaque in the center 7-8 minutes. Uncover and let cool. Break into large chucks.

Meanwhile, bring the broth to a boil in a small saucepan; reduced the heat and keep at a bare simmer.

Heat the oil in a large saucepan over medium heat. Add the onion and cook, stirring occasionally, until softened, about 4 minutes. Add the rice, garlic and the remaining ¾ tsp. of salt; cook constantly until the outer shell of the rice grains is translucent, about 1 minute.

Add one third (generous ¾ c.) of the hot broth and cook, stirring frequently, until absorbed, about 5 minutes. Repeat with another one third of the broth, stirring until absorbed before adding more. Add the remaining broth, the zucchini, and carrot; cook, stirring frequently, until the broth has been absorbed. Add the tomato, tomato-vegetable juice, and pepper; cook, stirring frequently, just until the rice and vegetables are tender about 5 minutes. Gently stir in the salmon and chives. Remove the pain from the heat and let stand, covered until the salmon is heated through, about 3 minutes. Serve at once.

Per Serving (1 1/2 c.) 372 CAL, 7 G FAT, 2 G SAT FAT, 0 G TRANS FAT, 56 MG CHOL, 1,096 MG SOD, 51 G CARB, 3 G FIB, 26 G PROT, 71 MG CALC.

# CREAMY STEAK DIJON

Prep 5 Min    Cook 15 Min          Serves 4

¾      lb. beef tenderloin, trimmed and cut into 1 ½ inch chunks
¾      tsp. salt
¼      tsp. black pepper
3      tsp. extra-virgin olive oil
1      (9-oz.) package sliced fresh cremini mushrooms
2      large shallots, minced
1 ½    c. reduced-sodium beef broth
1/3    c. fat-free sour cream
1      Tbsp. whole-grain Dijon mustard

Sprinkle the beef with ¼ tsp. of the salt and 1/8 tsp. of the pepper. Heat 2 tsp. of the oil in a 12-inch nonstick skillet over medium-high heat. Add the beef and cook, stirring, until browned and cooked through, about 4 minutes. Transfer to a large plate.

Heat the remaining 1 tsp. of oil in the skillet over medium-high heat. Add the mushrooms and the remaining ½ tsp. of salt and 1/8 tsp. of pepper, cook, stirring occasionally, until the mushroom start to release their liquid, about 1 minute. Add the shallots and cook, stirring frequently until the shallots are softened and the mushrooms are browned, about 3 minutes. Stir in the broth and bring to a boil. Cook until reduced by one half, about 6 minutes.

Stir in the beef and cook until heated through, about 1 minute. Remove the skillet from the heat; stir in the sour cream and mustard.

Per Serving (About 2/3 c.) 188 CAL, 9 G FAT, 3 G SAT FAT, 1 G TRANS FAT, 45 MG CHOL, 750 MG SOD, 7 G CARB, 1 G FIB, 19 G PROT, 47 MG CALC.

# FISH IN FOIL

| | |
|---|---|
| 1 | 8 oz. Can stewed tomatoes |
| ½ | c. steak sauce |
| 1 | clove garlic, minced |
| 4 | (4 oz. firm fish fillets) |
| 2 | c. frozen mixed vegetables |

In small bowl, combine stewed tomatoes, steak sauce, and garlic. Set aside.

Place each filet in center of double thickness foil; top each with filet with ½ cup mixed vegetables and ½ cup steak sauce mixture. Wrap foil securely.

Grill fish packets over medium heat 8-10 minutes or until fish flakes easily with fork. Serve immediately.

Makes 4 RSYL Servings

# LOW CALORIE MEAT MARINADES

It's important to keep the RSYL journey fun and easy. Change your meal plans frequently so you won't get bored. Here are some low calorie meat marinades that will add variety and space without lots of calories and/or fat.

# EASY TERIYAKI MARINADE

½ c. steak sauce
½ c. teriyaki sauce
2 tbs. Dijon Mustard
In small non-metal bowl combine above ingredients. Use to marinate beef, steak, poultry, or pork. Marinate for 1 hour before cooking. Makes ¾ cup.

# FLAVORFUL MARINADE

1 cube chicken or beef bouillon (low sodium) dissolved in water (follow package directions). Let chicken or beef marinate for 1 hour before cooking.

# MEXICAN CHICKEN STEW

Prep 5 MinutesCook 12 Minutes Serves 4

| | |
|---|---|
| 2 | c. reduced sodium chicken broth |
| 1 ½ | tsp. ground cumin |
| ¾ | c. instant brown rice |
| ¾ | lb. chicken tenderloins, cut into 1-inch chunks |
| 1 | (15 ½ oz) can black beans, rinsed and drained |
| 1 | (11 oz.) can Mexican-style corn, rinsed and drained |
| 1 ¼ | c. mild salsa |
| 3 | scallions, sliced |
| ½ | c. loosely packed fresh cilantro leaves, coarsely chopped |

Combine the broth and cumin in a Dutch oven and bring to a boil. Stir in the rice. Reduce the heat and simmer, covered, until the rice is partially cooked, about 3 minutes.

Stir in the chicken, beans, corn, salsa, and scallions; bring to a boil. Reduced the heat and cook, covered, stirring occasionally, until the rice and chicken are cooked through, 6-7 minutes. Sprinkle with the cilantro and serve.

Per Serving (1 ½ c.) 358 CAL, 4 G FAT, 1 G SAT FAT, 0 G TRANS FAT, 57 MG CHOL, 817 MG SOD, 51 G CARB, 13 G FIB, 31 G PROT, 117 MG CALC

# BLACK BEAN SOUP (VERY CREAMY, FILLING AND HIGH IN FIBER)

2        (15 ½ oz) cans Black Beans
½        cup Salsa
8 oz.    reduced fat low sodium chicken broth

Mix all ingredients together. This soup is excellent when prepared in a crock pot on low heat for 4 hours. This soup can also be made on the stove top. Bring all ingredients to a boil then lower heat and stir frequently. Heat through.

Serving suggestion: Serve with a spinach salad and flat bread.

## RSYL EASY DINNER IDEAS

What if you're cooking for one (or just a couple of people) and you don't have time to do a whole "recipe thing"? Try some of the menu options listed below. They are very easy - low in calories and fat. These are all things I ate while losing weight and that I continue to eat now.

## TURKEY BURGER

Grill or cook on stove (1 tsp extra virgin olive oil in pan) top 1 - 3 oz. lean turkey burger. Season to taste.

Serve with pita pocket lettuce, tomatoes, onions, pickles mustard and 2 - cups spinach salad. Dessert - fresh pineapple slices.

## TUNA PITA

3 oz Tuna (drained - packed in water) with 1 tsp fat free mayo on pita.

Serve with 1 c. of grapes and 1 serving of green beans.

# VEGGIE BURGER

3 oz veggie burger cooked in 1 tsp extra virgin olive oil. Season to taste. Serve with fat free feta cheese, spinach leaves, and sliced red onions.

# STRAWBERRY SPINACH SALAD

2 c. spinach leaves
Sliced red onion
½ c. sliced strawberries
1 tsp pine nuts
1 tsp fat free Feta cheese
Fat Free Raspberry vinaigrette dressing.

Mix together. Serve with dressing on the side.

This can be made ahead to make dinner preparation easier and faster.

# TURKEY GRAPE SALAD (VERY GOOD!!)

3 oz cubed turkey breast
1 c. grapes (halved)
2 tsp. Fat free may (mix all ingredients together and season to taste)
This can be made ahead to make dinner preparation easier and faster.

# RSYL FOOD TIPS ( IN NO PARTICULAR ORDER)

1) Never eat everything on your plate. (This is one time you don't have to listen to your mom).

2) Take small bites and chew slowly. (This is one time you should listen to your mom.

3) Drink 6 - 8 Servings of Water each day.

4) Eat the lowest calories foods on your plate first. This will help you eat less.

5) Keep a food journal. (Be honest and write everything down -

   I mean the whole truth and nothing but the truth).

6) Eat an AM and PM Snack of fresh fruits and/or vegetables every day.

7) Don't skip breakfast. (It really is the most important meal of the day).

8) Don't skip meals. You'll end up too hungry and be tempted to overeat.

9) Always keep healthy snacks close at hand. Keep a couple of healthy snacks in your car - at work - etc. That way if you're really hungry or tempted to eat if you've got a healthy option readily available.

10) Pray each day for the strength you need to RSYL.

# RSYL WORKOUT TIPS (IN NO PARTICULAR ORDER)

1) Always keep an extra workout bag in your car. That way you're always prepared.

2) Drink plenty of water as you work out. If you mouth gets dry while you're working out you have waited to long to re-hydrate.

3) Stretch before each workout. This will help you eliminate injury.

4) Don't overdo it. Your workout should challenge not "kill" you.

5) If you're new to working out - start with 3 - 4 days per week. Take it slowly   and build slowly.

6) If you're lifting weights - form is more important that the amount of weight. If you have to sacrifice form you are lifting too much weight.

7) You should always be able to talk while you are working out. If you are so out of breath that you cannot carry on a conversation - you are overdoing it.

8) If you have a trainer (and I recommend you do) follow their advice closely.

9) Choose a workout that you like. It doesn't matter whether it's walking, jogging, strength resistance training, aerobics, Pilates or whatever. Just select what you feel most comfortable doing and stick with it. Vary your workouts on occasion.

10) Avoid the on-again off-again work out. It's better to work out 3 days per week consistently than to work out 5 days one week and one day the next week.

***Read this list often. Many times it's the little things that get by us and cause us to get deterred.***

107

# RSYL - FAQ'S

*How do I get started?*

First get clearance to from a health professional to change your eating regime and also to embark on a fitness work out program.

After that, with the help of your health professional select a weight reduction nutritionally balanced eating program. I selected Weight Watchers. There are a number of weight reduction programs that are nutritionally sound for you to select from. Select what will work best for your lifestyle and work schedule. The good news is there are plenty of options.

*Do I have to work out?*

The short version of that answer is No. It may be of benefit to you though to consider working out. If you're open to working out and your health professional gives you clearance embarking on a reasonable fitness plan may help expedite your weight loss and assist you in becoming healthier.

The key for most people is to select something you enjoy. Walking is enjoyable for many people and it's easy on the joints. It can be done just about anywhere and you don't have to invest in any expensive equipment. For others, joining a fitness center and having a trainer help you may be the best way to start.

### *How often should I weigh?*

While you are RSYL weigh once per week. Weigh on the same day – about the same time – on the same scale. Now that I am in the maintenance phase I weigh every day. This helps me remind myself that I am doing okay. Do not weigh every day as you are losing weight – that becomes discouraging. While you are losing weight – weigh once per week. When you are in the maintenance phase you can continue to weigh once per week – or weigh every day. At that point it's up to you.

### *What do I do if I hit a plateau?*

Refer to the section in RSYL for information on breaking through a plateau. It can be done.

### *Do I have to starve?*

Absolutely not. It's not good for you. Many physicians and nutritionists also believe that starving shuts down your metabolism. That is not good when you're trying to lose weight. There are plenty of healthy foods to select from as you RSYL. Eat fresh vegetables and fruits. This will greatly assist you in not getting to hungry.

### *What are some tips for staying full?*

Drink 6 – 8 glasses of water per day. Plan healthy snacks throughout each day. Whether it's fresh fruit or vegetables eat a mid morning snack and an afternoon snack. You'll be surprised at how drinking more water and having two healthy snacks per day will assist you in staying full.

### *Will I ever be able to eat another cookie?*

Of course, when you are on the maintenance part of the RSYL journey you can enjoy occasional "treats". I can't imagine living my entire life without another cookie !!! The key thing is here it's on occasional cookie – not the whole box !!!

### Can I eat out?

Yes, you can eat out. It's important as you RSYL to be able to do things that you enjoy. Most of us can't live in isolation – nor should we want to. Just follow the section on right sizing your portions in this book. Also, consult with your weight loss program to find out the specific best options for you.

### What was your biggest challenge?

Learning to like fresh vegetables and fruits. It took me about the first 3 months of the RSYL journey. After about 3 months my taste buds started to change. Now I enjoy eating healthy foods. They taste good. Pray over every aspect of your RSYL journey.

### Do I have to eat Rabbit food?

RSYL is not about eating only rabbit food. God made lots of good food for His children to eat. There is a plethora of healthy foods to choose from.

### If I pray over my food will that stop me from gaining weight?

No. Not even if you try to "pray the calories or the fat out".

### What if I'm the only person in my family trying to RSYL?

That's a challenge I am well familiar with. When I went through my RSYL journey I was the only one in my house making the change. When all is said and done it is an individual journey and choice. Pray for the strength to make the changes. Over time it will get easier. The discipline you develop when you're the *"only one"* will assist you when you're out in the "real world". You will learn to eat what you want when you want – you won't be dependent on other people's food choices.

### What is BMI ?

Body Mass Index. Body mass index (BMI) is a formula that uses your weight and height to estimate your body fat and health risks. If your BMI is between 18.5 and 24.9, you're considered in a healthy weight range. *Source*:**MayoClinic.com.** Ask your trainer or healthcare professional to complete your BMI measurement. It is a very important tool in assessing your body/fat muscle ratio.

### What if I mess up on my food plan?

It's probably inevitable that at some point you'll go off of your food plan. Here's the thing do not listen to the lie that says: "I've already blown it so I should go ahead and eat the WHOLE thing". That's like saying I had a minor fender bender today so I think I'll go out and total my car on purpose.

No one (in their right mind) would say that. So if/when you go off your food plan do not make things worse. Smart people "cut their losses". Just get right back on your food plan. If you can work in some extra time at the gym - then do that. If not, just get back on the food plan. Record the incident in your food journal and then move forward and forget about it.

### What if I get bored with my workout ?

Most of us get bored if we do the same things the same way all of the time. The Right Sizing Your Life Journey is about making positive, healthy changes and that includes variety. If walking has become routine try cycling. If weight lifting has gotten into a routine - try some resistance training. The idea is to keep everything fresh. Plus most fitness experts concur that it's good to try different workouts and that it's the best way to burn fat. The concept is that things keep changing up so quickly your body doesn't know what to do so it starts burning fat. Make a concerted effort to try different things. This will keep your workout fresh, enjoyable and you'll receive the maximum benefits.

### Can I eat more if I workout?

Remember the idea here (when you're losing weight) is to burn more calories than you need. That's the only way to lose weight. Physical activity does burn calories and in some cases speed up our metabolism. The danger is to think you can eat a lot more just because you're working out and still lose weight. Take a look at the list below and see what kind of physical activity burns off how many calories.

| *Activity* * | *Burns Off* |
|---|---|
| **Ride Bike** (12 MPH) | 247 Calories |
| 29 Minutes | |
| **Shopping** | 241 Calories |
| 1 Hour 38 Minutes | |
| **Rollerblade** | 243 Calories |
| 18 Minutes | |
| **Hiking** | 243 Calories |
| 38 Minutes | |
| **Jumping Rope** | 128 Calories |
| 12 Minutes | |
| **Running** 2.3 Miles | 246 Calories |
| 23 Minutes | |
| **Raking Leaves** | 243 Calories |
| 53 Minutes | |
| **Horseback Riding** | 243 Calories |
| 57 Minutes | |
| **Yoga** | 120 Calories |
| 45 Minutes | |

**Packing for Vacation**          64 Calories

30 Minutes

**Chasing Kids @ Home**          120 Calories

28 Minutes

**Bobbi's Extreme Class**          1000 Calories

60 Minutes

* Based on 140 Pound Woman

As you can see working out can be a definite boost to your weight loss plan. Just make sure you're burning more calories than you're taking in to keep you in weight loss mode.

## SHOULD I TAKE VITAMINS?

If we lived in a perfect world all of our vitamins and minerals would come from our daily diet. Since we don't live in a perfect world taking vitamins can be a wise choice. Consult with your physician or nutritionist to find out what vitamins or supplements would best serve your dietary needs and goals.

These questions and more are covered in the Right Sizing Your Life 4 part DVD Conference series. To order your copy please visit www.monicaspeaks.com

# RSYL INSPIRATION

When you're tired of the food plan, working out and drinking water--just take some time to relax and receive a blessing from God's Word. It's our all important power source and God's Word has the ability to Right Size your life. His Word is nourishment for a weary, hungry soul and will give you a fresh perspective when nothing else will work.

Romans 8:28 NLT

"And we know that God causes everything to work together for the good of those who love God and are called according to his purpose for them."

Matthew 7: 7- 10 NLT

"Keep on asking, and you will receive what you ask for. Keep on seeking, and you will find. Keep on knocking, and the door will be opened to you.   For everyone who asks, receives. Everyone who seeks, finds. And to everyone who knocks, the door will be opened. "You parents—if your children ask for a loaf of bread, do you give them a stone instead?  Or if they ask for a fish, do you give them a snake? Of course not!"

John 15: 16 – 27 NLT

"You didn't choose me. I chose you. I appointed you to go and produce lasting fruit, so that the Father will give you whatever you ask for, using my name. This is my command: Love each other."

Philippians 4: 8 NLT

"And now, dear brothers and sisters, one final thing. Fix your thoughts on what is true, and honorable, and right, and pure, and lovely, and admirable. Think about things that are excellent and worthy of praise."

Hebrews 13:8 NLT

"Jesus Christ is the same yesterday, today, and forever."

Luke 5:31 NLT

"Jesus answered them, "Healthy people don't need a doctor—sick people do. [32] I have come to call not those who think they are righteous, but those who know they are sinners and need to repent."

Matthew 11: 28 NLT

Then Jesus said, "Come to me, all of you who are weary and carry heavy burdens, and I will give you rest.

Matthew 18:19 NLT

"I also tell you this: If two of you agree here on earth concerning anything you ask, my Father in heaven will do it for you.

2 Thessalonians 2:16 NLT

Now may our Lord Jesus Christ himself and God our Father, who loved us and by his grace gave us eternal comfort and a wonderful hope, [17] comfort you and strengthen you in every good thing you do and say."

Made in the USA
San Bernardino, CA
16 May 2015